Dating for Men

The Ultimate Guide to Approach and Attract Your Ideal Woman - Includes How to Text and How to Talk to Women

Sabrina Schuman

Table of Contents

How to Text a Woman

Discover How a Girl Wants You to Text Her even If You're Shy and Never Run Out of Things to Say

Sabrina Schuman

Introduction

S o you have exchanged numbers or social media with a girl. Now what?

Most guys get too caught up on random bullshit texting rules the dating community has made up. The PUA's say you should wait 24 hours to text the girl, you shouldn't put emojis, and your text should contain perfect grammar, etc. It's all bullshit.

It doesn't matter if you take 24 hours to text her or 24 minutes. The fact is she will get the text either way. It's what you text that is more important. My personal preference is to text a girl after 7pm. This is when people aren't usually busy. If you text a girl throughout the day, expect her to reply late since people are busiest throughout the day. They go to work, they do their groceries, they might go to the gym, etc.

I wouldn't recommend texting a girl on a Friday or Saturday night because most women go out on these days. If you text her on a Friday night, you are subconsciously saying, "I have nothing better to do on a Friday night, so I am texting you." If you really want to text her on a Friday night for whatever reason, I recommend you start the conversation off with "I am at this club and..." or "I'm getting ready to go out ...". This shows that you aren't sitting alone at home waiting for her to text back like a needy guy.

Purpose of Texting

The main purpose of texting is not to have a long deep conversation with the girl. The only purpose of texting is to get the woman out on a date. If you're in high school, then sure, text the girl and try to have a conversation with her over text, but if you're a man, you should use texting to get her out. Leave the conversation to when you meet up.

This doesn't mean, however, that your second text should be you setting up a date. You shouldn't start a conversation; you should, however, tease and be flirty with her through text. This will give her all the positive emotions she needs to agree to meet up with you. More on that later.

The First Text

Many guys stress over the first text and sit there endlessly thinking of the perfect first text. The first text is the most important. If the girl is attractive, then you are most likely not the only guy texting her. You are most likely the only non-needy guy texting her. You must send a low investment text that doesn't end in a question mark to show that you aren't like all the other needy guys. What do I mean by low investment text?

A low investment text is a simple text which you didn't have to put a lot of thought into. You don't have to send the "perfect text."

Avoid asking a question in the first text. Instead, text a statement. If your first text has a question mark in the end, then the girl will feel obligated to text back. If, however you send her a simple statement, she can choose to ignore it. This is a perfect way to see if the girl is interested or not.

There are times where a girl will ignore your text even if you had a great interaction. When this happens, guys get confused as to why they do this. The reason is because of their emotional drives. Have you experienced a scenario where you are texting a girl, and she takes a while to reply to your text, but once you are in an argument with her, her replies are almost instant? This is because of her emotional drive.

When you were interacting with a girl, you would have given her positive emotions and kept her interested. The next day, though, when you text her, her emotions might be flat. If they are, she won't feel the urge to text you back and will probably forget to text you later. Even if she had the best interaction with you last night, if she isn't feeling it, she won't text you back.

There are also texts that you should not send. The worst one is "Hey, it's John from the bar last night. I was wearing a red shirt, remember me?". This is the neediest text you could possibly send the girl. Sure it seems sweet and innocent, and you might be thinking if she was drunk the night before, she might not have remembered you, but this text screams, "Give me validation." Instead, you should send your statement or a reference to something you talked about in your interaction and then just add your name at the end.

Instagram

If you are going to text a girl through Instagram or other social media, you have the advantage of sending photos and videos. You can always start the conversation by sending her a funny photo.

Sometimes I like to send a funny 4-second video. I have a specific video I send which always makes me, and everyone I show it to, laugh. You can be sure the girl laughed at the video if she replies. Not only does sending a funny video separate me from all the other guys it also gives her positive emotions that she associates with me. If you're stuck, find a short funny video and send her that.

When she is scrolling through her DM's, all she is going to see is needy text messages from guys, and then she will see your message "sent a photo." Women are curious; she will click on it.

Once she laughs, you have just given her positive emotions no other guy has given her on a first text. What is lower investment than a simple funny photo? Again she doesn't have to reply to it, but I bet you she will.

Waiting

When I first started getting women's numbers. I would text them and would just wait. What I have not known at the time is that waiting is the worst possible thing you can do. I would start to overthink and become very negative: "The girl isn't interested," "She is probably talking to other guys," etc.

When you have sent your first text, don't just sit there and wait for a text back. Even if you have been talking for a while, you shouldn't wait for any girl's text back. You need to realize that she has a life too. She could still be at work, in the gym, cooking, at a family gathering, shopping, having a shower, eating, reading, her phone is on mute, driving. There are a million different reasons that may be holding her back from replying to you.

The worst possible thing you could do that will let her lose all her attraction towards you is to keep bombarding her with needy messages until she replies. "Why are you not replying?" "Are you there?" "Why are you ignoring me" etc. These kinds of texts

15

subconsciously tell her, "I have no other women in my life, so I am going to sit here on my phone waiting for you to reply because I have nothing better to do." That doesn't sound very attractive, does it?

Instead, what the attractive man does is goes out and has fun. He lives his life. He doesn't spend hours waiting for a girl he has talked to for an hour to reply to his message. He pursues his hobbies and passion; he reads a book, watches a film, spends time with family and friends, and many more, instead of staring at his phone waiting for a text message that will give him validation.

Now that you know what to text, it is important to know what you shouldn't do when texting a girl.

Paragraphs

If the majority of texts on the screen are coming from you, it shows that you are way more invested than she is. One-sided texting is when you are sending paragraphs and she texting back a one-line text. It shows that you are putting so much effort into starting a conversation with her, but she isn't reciprocating that effort.

If you find yourself sending paragraphs, try to hold back a little and let her invest a bit. Slowly decrease the amount of text you send. Remember, you aren't trying to have a long conversation with her. You are purely trying to get her to meet up with you.

Don't Text Her Every Day

Give her some space. The reason women rarely give out their numbers is to not get bombarded with texts every day, 24/7. Don't text her for a day; give her some space after you have had a little back and forth texting. You give her a chance to miss you even slightly. If you are free to text her every single day 24/7 is says something about how interesting your life is.

Calling

I am not a big fan of calling women. Many guys have success by doing this because it adds a new depth to the interaction. It is better to hear someone's voice rather than read their texts. However, the reason I don't call is that it is a too high-pressure situation for a girl. She could be very insecure and not pick up the phone because "Her voice doesn't sound good" or some bullshit excuse. I know a girl that won't pick up the phone unless she is wearing make-up. The girl might not even have time to talk to you on the phone.

My advice is if the conversation through text is going amazingly and you have both been replying pretty fast, then I suggest you ask her if it's cool to call her first. She won't be hit with that element of surprise and put the phone down because of the pressure. Use a time restriction too.

"I'm going to call you real quick because I don't want to text" or just give her any reason whatsoever. Wait for her to reply "Sure," and then you just call her. During texting, your main purpose is to get her out on a date. When talking on the phone, however, you have the opportunity to have a great conversation since her replies will be instant. After your conversation, you set up the date.

Setting Up a Date

You have been texting back and forth or talking on the phone, and everything is going great. You want to go on a date with this girl.

Asking the girl out may seem slightly intimidating at first, but over time, you will overcome your fear of setting up dates.

While you are texting the girl, you will want to make sure you have given her some positive emotions by either teasing and flirting with her or making her laugh. You will then send a text message saying, "What are you doing later?" or "What are you doing Wednesday night?". Her reply will be similar to one of two replies.

She will either reply with a plan she has set up for later, or she will reply with "Nothing."

If she replies with "I'm going to the cinema later," she is either actually going to the cinema, or she is making up an excuse for you not to ask her out. Either way, don't get butt hurt; you can always try again in a few days. Stay in a positive mood. You don't have to completely end all interactions between you and the girl because she didn't agree to go out with you once.

If, however, her reply is "Nothing," that means she is expecting you to ask her out, and you should do it immediately. Remember, you need to show your dominance. Just like when exchanging numbers, you should never ask the girl out on a date. Instead, say, "Let's grab a coffee Wednesday night." If she agrees, then you can work out the details.

You need to show that you don't go on a date with any woman. You do this by adding a statement that will make her qualify herself. All you have to do is say, "Only if you're cool" or "As long as you don't turn out to be a psycho."

The final text should look like this:

"Let's grab coffee Wednesday night, as long as you don't turn out to be a psycho."

You can see that you qualifying the girl takes the pressure off the situation. If you say, "Do you want to go on a date on Wednesday?" this puts too much pressure on her. With the text above, you show dominance and also take the pressure of her.

There is much more to learn. Keep on reading.

Please note that when I use the word "girl," most of the time, I am referring to a grown woman unless I am speaking in the contest of high school.

Chapter 1:

Set Your Mindset for Success

The question of attraction and seduction depends on the mindset that one has. The mindset, in this case, relates to how one views themselves and others. In essence, one needs to acquire a mentality that will put one in the position to understand himself in relation to the environment around him. This is by having an accurate understanding of yourself, your abilities, and weaknesses. Based on this, you can then begin to figure out how you can use these abilities to influence the environment around you and to make interactions directing them towards your desired objective.

The mindset of a person who wants to be a phenomenal seducer but has been bad at it is that they view themselves as having something wrong in their personality. They think they have a weakness that makes it difficult for them to either draw attraction or get women to acquire a liking for them. They are probably reading this book with the hope that this weakness gets fixed. They believe there is probably some secret formula that one has to use in approaching women and talking to them in order to be successful in seduction.

They also look for validation and think that they have to have women in order to be "conquerors." They do not feel self-sufficient and hence seek to desperately woo women in order to appear cool in the eyes of people. It is as if seduction is a means of proving that they can do this probably better than anyone. Yet when they try it, they fail miserably and hence going back to self-doubt mode.

The thing is, seduction newbies are generally wannabes who are motivated by a wrong mindset. They fall short in the mentality, and hence they cannot be successful with women. They try to be fake by trying the popular methods that peers talk about or the ones they see in the movie. They think that covers up on what they are, yet in reality, they failed at the most important step; the mindset.

The reality is if you view yourself as having weaknesses, whether imagined or real, you make them a reality. You feel limited, and no matter what you do to overcome them, the reality of this thought does not let you be free. Successful people do not entertain a thought that they are inadequate or incomplete. Perhaps because thinking like this does not help. You do not fix yourself, and it is not even tested that fixing yourself will lead to better results. Whatever you perceive as being your nature, you start to become. Better have a positive self-concept, it will call out the best in you, and you probably will feel better about yourself and reduce limitations that can come from the mind.

It is vital to avoid the thought that there is a secret formula for handling women. There is none, as this just flows in the same vein in reinforcing negative self-concept. It makes you jealous. You feed the belief that there is something wrong with you and that success with women requires some magical forces that others have and which you have to get out and acquire. Understand that seduction happens naturally, and you only need to package yourself with the right mindset in order to either trigger it or accurately identify where you can be successful. Attraction is also something natural among people, and sometimes you are focused so much on formulas and thinking about your weaknesses that you cannot realize when an attraction is occurring. Sometimes, men only have to learn how to deal with attraction when it comes their way. Some men become nervous and start following certain formulas and applying routines and rules on every occasion of attraction. If there was a secret formula with seduction, then perhaps so many men would have a dynasty of lovers since using the formula guarantees you success with the woman. However, there is no man who is too excellent with seduction to win every woman that is an object of his lust. Get that out of your mind and know you can evoke attraction as you are, just with a few refinements of your random advances.

Correct Your Mindset

There are no tips that one should purport to give you when it comes to how you handle women. What you need is the ability to be socially intelligent. This is because attraction occurs naturally, and it is not so much something that requires you to fix yourself. You are complete the way you are, and you only need to use what you have in you to make it work for you. What works, for now, may not work tomorrow. Just go through a process of social intelligence.

Social intelligence is just the way you interact in a way that makes your presence memorable. This is by behaving in a manner that makes a woman feel an urge to get closer to you. You must be able to enchant and cause a woman to feel she is special and set apart from others. That means that your interactions should be quite purposeful, although not predictably so. Just learn how to behave, to look, to converse, and to connect.

Learn how women open up to you in a way to give you a chance and how they show rejection. Know how to capitalize on chances through social intelligence. These are all subject to how you interact and what you say. If you are texting, having social intelligence is what will guide you in how you socialize in the online space. Know how to lead a girl in the direction of your advances and have the ability to read signals and adjust or even retreat. Do not be rigid and fixated. Do not have an egotistic mindset that tells you that you must win. Do not try to induce things when they seem to be stuck. When a woman does not seem attracted to you, do not be compelling; hover in the region you are at, applying conscious self-awareness until she opens up to another region or level of interaction. Sometimes, women do not like men the first time. This is due to preconceptions, past experiences, and stereotyping.

You, therefore, do not just show up with your haircut and expect that every woman will be swept off the feet. While it may have been the thing that tipped the balance in your favor on one woman, it may just remind another woman of another man who had similar characteristics and is the biggest regret of her life. That is why seduction and attraction are about learning to let things unfold.

However, understand that as much as there are men who have been famed for having a lot of affairs and who swim in covet of women, no one is universally likable. Do not think that there is something you are going to learn, and then you emerge and make a series of kills and begin to be so successful with seduction. As intimated earlier, there are people whom you naturally piss off, and they even just hate you, and that is naturally occurring just as attraction is natural. It, therefore, does not matter much what you learn in order to make yourself the most seductive man around.

So, What Matters?

You can never be the person that understands what every woman thinks. You have no intelligence to grasp what every woman has gone through in their life just by meeting them. It is possible to understand certain common patterns in the behavior of women, but that does not include comprehending the workings in the minds of a woman that make her see you in the way that she does. Definitely, therefore, you need to be real and not fake it as you are not bound to even correct the way a woman perceives you, even if you say things that fool her.

Additionally, seduction should not impede the fact that it is a natural phenomenon. This means that one should not try to be manipulative or make a fool out of the woman. This only makes you less attractive, and manipulation only evokes hate that is momentarily hidden behind the attraction. Do not try to make a woman start to think you are this when you are that. Fooling her just to take advantage of her or lay her is the greatest demonstration of self-doubt. It is a show that you do not think you can win by being what you are. There is no worse statement of self-doubt than acting to be something that you are not. You cannot be loved when you even cannot love yourself.

Understand Seduction

Women naturally have the disposition of acting like they are disinterested. They will want to appear like they do not like something when they do. That is why seduction is necessary. Seduction is when you use various advances to make the woman finally agree with herself to be involved with the person she deeply knows she wanted to be involved with. This comes through creating a connection that is real. It is about boldly showing who you are and letting her decide that you are just what she wanted. You do not fool, you do not fake it, you tell her subconscious that you are this kind of a man and appeal to it to accept and desire you.

This means that knowing who you truly are is the most important thing that matters. Your mindset should be aware of who you are, and in pursuit to learn how to seduce and attract, it should be a pursuit to understand and get to a comprehensive acceptance of who and what you are. This is what is referred to as finding the self. It is the precise and natural way that seduction goes. That a man, as he is, goes up to a woman and tells her that he wants to mate with her. She then decides to pair with the man or turn it down. It all is in the power of the woman to choose. Or otherwise, it will not be seduction but being forceful. Your part as a man is learning how to model your true self and present it to the woman.

This being the case, one needs to fix one's mindset on what really matters. Think about being the best with presenting your true self. Focus on the only thing that is reliable and which is to be real. The woman will have to deal with it, and you will start to realize just how okay you are. You will realize that you suppressed a lot of excellence and success trying to be what you are not. In creating a great mindset of success, you have to question yourself on various aspects that define you and lead you to discover who you are. The essence of doing this is to know what the girls deal with when you are presenting yourself to them. You will be able to realize sometimes why some girls reject you and what others have difficulty dealing with your kind. Knowing yourself will also help to cut your expectations of how women receive you to size.

When you know who and what you are, you can clearly know what can work and who can deal with you and who is bound to have problems dealing with you and what you are. It will help in ensuring that you direct your efforts to seduce people who are open are likely to be open to you. Not everyone can deal with you, and it can be a show of extravagant expectation to think that everyone has the power to handle you. Go through the process of self-discovery, and you will also learn how to know what kind of a woman she is.

How to Know Who You Are

In the end, make what you want and your aspirations a part of who you are. This is by presenting a persona that is ambitious and which is in the process of transformation. For instance, if you are a sportsman, believe that you are a champion and train in a way that a sportsman does. Handle your issues in life like a sportsman, and that is what women will perceive. Just like Mohammed Ali from the age of 19 regarded himself as the world's greatest, view yourself as a champion, a conqueror, or important. This will build your persona and will elevate you from the levels of pettiness. It will also call out the best from you, and hence you will present the real you in a way that the woman can overlook your downsides. That is the mindset of success, and it will make you do well socially even as you excel in seduction and attraction.

Chapter 2:

How to Text Women Online

B ut before the date is set and you start to flirt on a text, it is necessary to know how to start texting her on social media or after getting her number; this is the first approach. The main thing when texting women you just met is that texting isn't good for types of conversations that "get to know you." Leave such conversations for when you're still together. It is because the words you use are the least important thing in a conversation; the predominant feature is your body language and your tone of voice, and those are absent when you're writing.

During texts, flirt a little and keep it light—a little bit of banter. Don't worry about using emoticons, which lets her know you're playing and messing around. One way to increase attraction is to bring up something the two of you connected over when you met. Jokes work best for this because they put her in a fun and playful space right away.

After the first approach to text and after bantering your way to a healthy level of confidence and friendship, you want to concentrate the conversation on making plans. After all, you weren't asking for her phone number so that the two of you could endlessly sit there, talking. Talk to her about things for which you two share a passion, then plan to go out and do something together. If she is not involved at first, don't worry: she might like you, but not the plans, or she may have something to do legitimately. But if she's shooting down ideas repeatedly, then you're probably better off moving on. Either she is not as into of you as you think, or she has no time to date.

Once you both decide to go on a date, the discussion will turn to logistics entirely; keep it simple, plain and fun. When you have decided on the specifics, such as what you're doing, where, when, and how you're both getting there, you can go back to flirting. Perhaps, the last thing you want to talk about is what you watched on TV or what your childhood was like. For an in-person conversation, there is much to say. Avoid the long conversations about your favorite TV shows and what you think about the job for when you see each other.

How to Start Texting?

The first text should be an introduction rather than going forward with a very generic "hi" text. The first important step is to have a special and exciting introduction. Words can be your friend as well as your enemy. One of the main ways that most guys screw up big time is how they approach. Such guys often start with a "hello or hi" text to play it safe, and that is the reason there is no response. Women yearn for passion and desire. If you want to create a desirable self-image with less, you should be able to say more. Many guys try to break the ice, one which may never have been there! I think it is clear enough that your first text depends very much on the level of interconnection between you two.

Let's take two examples of this:

"Princess, hey …."

Or

"Hi, Lovely …."

As you can clearly see, these texts are perfect if you are in a serious relationship or are close enough to tease her. However, if you send these texts to a woman who has not yet got a good understanding of you and your character, you are doomed to flag or fail.

Remember, you're aiming to build passion, desire, and appeal. In other words, the guy should strive to introduce himself elegantly, avoid at all costs stupid phrases and/or openers, and start small talk to build relationships.

Here is one more professional approach:

"Hi (NAME), it was great (experience) ...."

Or

"Hi (NAME), that was a blast yesterday! I was thinking ......"

In many circles, it is believed that starting a text with her name could yield better results.

Since not many do that, the person doing it stands out quickly. This is, not to mention, a very elegant way to introduce yourself, and it doesn't seem weird.

Go for a conversation from here. A great suggestion is to remind her of the event you both experienced in some way- let's say it was a party or concert (Hey Tiffany, the concert was great! I can't believe you did ...). It is very important that a person writes one, maybe two lines, from one to two short sentences, and wait for an answer. Do not make it look needy, and definitely avoid filling the entire chat page with your text messages.

The thing under consideration is the fact that a guy shouldn't spend too much time texting the girl. Remember the event; the guy should ask her if she'd enjoyed it, say next week there's a similar activity going on, and ask her to join him. Something similar might just do the job well. Put in a few more phrases to make it sound like a real little chat about text and then ask her. Try nothing too fancy because the more a person writes, the greater chances of screwing things up.

Women are full of emotion. They are much more emotional than the guys. If you want to grasp a woman's art of messaging, it would be your best bet to bind her to you, to make her emotionally addicted.

The most effective way of attracting and connecting with women is by:

- Sending her funny texts-helps; you break the ice and get the conversation going
- Callback Humor can help you to connect to her in a relatively simple and effective way
- Making her happy-making her emotionally addicted, and attracted to you

First, find something funny and text it to her. If you've got something as easy as a post or GIF or maybe a video and you think it could impress her, go for it. It's a different approach from pickup lines, but it will provoke a new response from her because she never expected it.

The second approach is the "Callback Humor" This simply means referring to the thing you mentioned when you first met her. If you talked about animals and she said she will do anything for little kittens, it's good to send her something about cats. Not only is this something she loves and enjoys, but the chances of getting her text you back are very good.

The last, and the most effective way, is to create the emotions inside her. The guy has to figure out what text can make a woman smile. It is not the same as humor on callback. It is much stronger than that. Indeed, a great tactic would be to start with something that you spoke about at the initial meeting and then apply this step.

To text a girl, you must figure out funny things. However, the goal is not merely to laugh at something dumb and pointless. The main idea will be the filling of the environment with joy and enthusiasm to make her feel more relaxed around. It can be a means to learn how to carry on a conversation over text. In addition, she'll get closer and more attracted to you.

Pickup Lines

Pick (someone) up has been used as slang to have a casual sexual encounter with a person since at least the 17th century. The slang inspired the "pickup" adjective, used to describe a line or rehearsed remark, used to strike up a conversation with a person for romantic or sexual pursuance.

One such instance of pickup line was used in 1979 to describe a line of dialog in the classic 1969 movie Midnight Cowboy when the main character tells a wealthy lady: "Beg pardon, ma'am, I'm new town here, just in from Houston, Texas, and looking for the Statue of Liberty."

The term pickup line spread throughout the 1980s and by the 1990s had become associated with the unadvised efforts of men to talk to women in bars (e.g., "Did it hurt when you fell from heaven?"). Usually, pickup lines start with a question followed by a punch line (for example, "Do I know you? Because you look like my next girlfriend.").

Upon the advent of social media and online dating in the 2000s, pickup lines spread across digital communication. They take the form of a private or direct message to someone on these social media platforms, aiming to draw their attention in setting up a date or talking further.

Mistakes to Avoid

There are some mistakes that a person should avoid as they end up complicating the chances for a date.

- Too Nervous

It matters not if this is your first attempt, or perhaps the tenth that you asked this week. You'll feel somewhat insecure and indecisive about texting for a date or call. This is a common problem in the Arena of Dating. So, if you notice that you're getting nervous and impulsive, the best thing you can do would be to leave the phone, take a few minutes of deep, slow breathing, perhaps drink some water and try to clear your mind. Although this may not take away all the anxiety, it will surely put you in a better position not to screw things up.

- Texting a Girl the Same Day after She Gave the Number

You can do that, of course, but be cautious. Don't try to hurry stuff up. It would be better to ask for a drink or something. Don't rush through the dating process. You go after an emotional attachment, and this is only built up in the long run.

- Texting the Girl's Number after Two Weeks

Even if you feel like you've really been able to connect with her and build the foundation of a relationship, if you write her one or two weeks later, you'll find out that the passion is dead.

- Do not Over-Text

Text ideas are to provoke curiosity and take her out on a date and not a forum for discussion. In fact, the more you're writing to her, the greater her chance of seeing you as a texting buddy and not as a potential future boyfriend.

- Speaking of Her as a Guy

That's exactly how you're supposed to text a girl once you've got her number, like a man and not a woman. The thing that surprises people is how softly most people seem to converse in person as well as face to face. You're the man; you're supposed to be the boss, the one with confidence, the alpha male talking his talk and walking his walk. Nonetheless, from observations, no one behaves like that next to someone.

Double-check your grammar and spelling, for example. No girl worth dating will be interested in a guy who can't even write an entire sentence right. Then, be a little better. Being sweet, loving, and compassionate is one thing, and not being able to stand up for yourself and agree with all that is happening to you is a whole other.

- Don't pay Attention to Her

The girl is there to "fill a gap" in your life and not to make it in it. Some people might have a hard time understanding it, but you have your own life and responsibilities. And you have to pay attention to them.

Don't text her constantly. This way, you say directly that you don't have anything going on in your life, and you're thinking about her all day. This ends up with her being more distant and avoids replying to your texts. It is one thing to give the attention needed and another to be obsessed with her like a creep.

- Useful Compliments

A good compliment can secure a home run for you, while a bad one may break your chances in a moment. You should stick to a casual way of talking. Especially if this is your first text since you were given her number, avoid compliments, especially as initial text conversation openers.

It is important to note that compliment has the whole purpose of being sudden, provoking, and sounding genuine.

- Copy Her Style

If you wonder about an appropriate way to email her, you can do the easiest thing, just mimic her style of writing. You may want to mirror the way she interacts with you in order to share the same atmosphere.

- Being Too Sexual

It would be a bad idea to over-sexualize the conversation. Now, a thin line exists between what you can do and what is acceptable. In reality, women love teasing. It is all good to be playful while still being able to provoke passion and emotion, even lust.

There should really be a sort of connection between the two of you, which should be both physical and mental. This is what real relationships are built on, after all.

Nevertheless, guys mistakenly overdo the talking or, in this case, texting in their attempts to carry the message.

Telling her a dirty joke or something of that sort is one thing and totally different from flirting with her always. When she gets the impression that you are only interested in her because you want to use her for your own satisfaction, then your chances suddenly drop to nil.

- Going Across the Board

Even if you think you've planned and organized everything and everything falls perfectly in line, there's always a risk that maybe she'll be busy, maybe she won't want to date you, or she doesn't have any feelings towards you. Both of these circumstances are normal and can happen. Therefore you have to pay close attention to what you say and do.

If your plan hasn't worked out for some reason and you are being rejected, just say something like "All is fine" and get off your phone right away. Do not pressure her in the chat or badmouth or ask her to go out with you.

The fact that she now doesn't want to go out with you doesn't necessarily mean she won't go out in the future with you. It clearly shows you need to develop more emotional appeal before you can take her out.

Chapter 3:

The Approach

T he correct strategy of approaching women remains a contentious issue for men to date. As such, it is not clear which methods are the most effective and which aren't. This is because of relatively split opinions on the matter. Some people deem the direct approach as the most effective and claim the indirect approach is evasive and time-wasting. Others support the indirect approach where the man usually hides his intentions in disguised behavioral manifestations towards the woman and appears as if he is not even out to hit on her at all. It is therefore important to explore these approaches for purposes of comparison.

Direct Method

This method is usually coming out and declaring your intentions to hit on a woman in no uncertain terms. The proponents of this approach think that it is the most effective and ensures time is not wasted. They also feel that it does not dig so much into one's dating abilities and can be affected by anyone. They claim that the indirect method only raises a buffer that makes it impossible for one to progress his advances at the girl.

Whenever you come out and try to engage a girl in a conversation, she is not daft as not to start analyzing you. Even if you claim to have misdirected a text, she will have to analyze it, and she perceptively can already tell that you probably are approaching her.

There indeed are girls who are oblivious and do not even realize what the man is up to and only end up finding themselves victims of circumstances. However, when you act like you are not interested in her, she probably is aware of it the whole time and can think of you as being pansy.

With this approach, it is required if a man to be clear about his intentions and purpose to be impressive from the first minute. That as a man, you get out and have a glow on you that can naturally evoke admiration and trigger desire from the woman. If it is texting, use every opportunity she allows you from the first minute to be purposeful and to impress. Do not engage in idle texting with a girl as she will only relegate you further into a place where you will not be able to break through to her again.

Those supporting this approach feel a woman should not be allowed a lot of time to know your vulnerabilities and weaknesses before you already have won her over. That immediately you encounter her and decide that she is worth hitting on, you gauge the chances of how she will receive you. Once your perception tells you that she is open to you, do not go beating around the bush. She will also show you already whether she wants you to go on. That this will save you a lot of moments of uncertainty and possibly make you lose your chances in case she is taken by another swift guy while you continue buying time engaging in false disinterest.

The reason why men can be afraid of this approach is the fact that they fear rejection. They, therefore, want to coil around and find a way of being accepted completely. However, using this approach assumes that nothing you do can change the girl's mind about you if you have not impressed the first time. That the first impression determines how the girl will perceive you for the longest time, and you can have a hard time changing that. If she shows some interest and allows you close to her, it is supposed to be taken advantage of no matter what the result will be. If she is not into your advances, waiting will not help it. You will only be delaying the rejection, and hence you will not realize the worth of having waited.

There is some degree of defiance with the people who use this strategy. They are undeterred by rejection, particularly because if it is online, it is a girl they do not know. They have no time to play games and idly engage in purposeless talks. The man goes straight to the point and clearly shows that he is out to hit on her. If the girl does not buy it, they move on to the next girl they are texting.

Besides, some girls detest insincerity and acting out. She may like you for all the reasons and hate you for not being able to stand up to yourself and tell yourself to go out and get what you want. They may associate it with an unstable personality, and if she likes you so much, she may make it difficult for you to ever approach her. So you will be kept in a friendship zone, or if it is texting, she may not allow you to get her to a meet-up. She thinks you are not confident and have a lot of self-doubts which is an anti-seducer and a show of weakness that may just not be what she is looking for in the man.

This approach, however, does not apply to everyone at all. Particularly for texting a girl, it may work, but in very few circumstances. You should not be too forward with your intentions in such a way that you overwhelm her. A girl has got to be allowed time to express herself and understand why she is wanted. Besides, some girls may deem it rude and think you have a compromised perception of who they are. She may be interested, but she may think you are making her appear cheap. It, therefore, still requires you to be perceptive and understand the girl you are going out to.

If it is a girl you have a history of and who has any idea of who you are, it will probably work when you are direct. Assume it is a girl you have been coincidentally meeting on several occasions in the commuter train and have been doing some non-verbal communication; she may have some preparedness. You could walk up to her and ask for her number.

You can then go straight to the point here. You will text her and introduce yourself. You could then straight away ask about a possible evening out since you already have an idea what time she is out of work, and you are sure she should be just about able to make it.

Another advantage of this approach, aside from simply saving time and the trouble, is what it makes the girl think of you. It somehow comes out as a typical masculine expression, and while it may come out rough, the girl may feel you are confident and sure. It is also a bold expression of desire that the girl feels quite flattered for. That you walked across the street and stood up to her to say she is attractive is deeply complementing. Chances are that she has not had that happen to her before, and she may not going to have it happen to her so many times in her life. So on a text message, you can also be that abrupt but careful because she has no idea of who you are. However, texting her for the first time and saying that you could not hold it back and that there is no better time, place, or platform to let her know how you find her attractive will get her thinking.

However, it is also disadvantageous, as already explained earlier. It is a high risk even when its rewards are equally high.

Indirect Approach

This approach is used by a lot of men, particularly given the risks that are associated with the direct approach. In this approach, the man lays low and, in some instances, sends mixed signals. It has already been mentioned that being direct can make you shoot yourself in the foot and bring to an unprecedented what would have been a promising interaction with a girl. When using this approach, the goal is to create a basis for the attraction between you. Sometimes, women may not directly get attracted to a man until time has passed.

For instance, you hear a new song played on the radio, and you do not think it is great. Then you listen to it the second time it is played, and you still do not understand why the song you don't even like has to still be on air. Then you later go out for a karaoke night. Then the song is sung, and you find yourself up and jamming to it alongside other people.

That is how attraction also works. It may not happen immediately but can be evoked with familiarity. Some of the reasons that ladies do not like men are because of the preconceptions they have. When a man is dressed in a certain way, the girl initially thinks that he not interesting and exciting. Going to her at this stage is bound to attract a rebuff. However, take time, let her interact with you, and discover that the exact opposite is true. What is ever so good with women is when their preconceptions are challenged. If she thought the man to be a bore and the man becomes quite exciting, she feels more drawn to him.

As a man, I take it that you are supposed to have a plan on how to handle a woman. This should involve planning and strategizing, and that means you need an approach that will allow you to execute the plan. This will minimize the risks and help you plan, reposition and ensure you are quite accurate.

Chapter 4:

How to Get Her Number

Y ou've been talking a few minutes, and she seems like she's into you. But will she give you her phone number? Will she go out with you?

First of all, you need to be in the mindset that, of course, she will. She has given you no reason to think she wouldn't, so keep that positivity.

You have to believe that every woman you are interested in will give you her number. It's not arrogance. It's just a feeling of positivity and abundance. You are an intelligent, good-looking, and interesting guy, so there is no reason she would not want to get to know you. If you operate on this level, you will radiate confidence.

So, how do you move the conversation to a point where you can get her number?

Small Talk to Real Conversation

The biggest trick to moving from small talk and casual conversation to something more meaningful is to validate their interests and pull them into a deeper conversation.

What all this means is: find the small things in what they are saying or doing that can be seen as important by both of you.

Let's try a hypothetical situation:

You are at a coffee shop, and you notice a beautiful woman waiting for her coffee right next to you. You give her a smile; she smiles back, and you have some good eye contact. She comments on your shirt color, and you thank her.

Right as your coffee comes, you notice she has a nice bracelet that is very unique. You comment that it's really cool. She smiles, thanks you, and says she got it when she was traveling in Asia. You say that sounds cool, and she smiles, says goodbye, and leaves.

What happened?

You had the perfect opportunity to turn casual small talk into a much deeper conversation. She gave you the perfect opening when she said she got her bracelet in Asia.

That's the opportunity to take a bit of small talk information and turn it into a conversation that is meaningful. Travel is a perfect opportunity. When people take a trip, especially to another country or part of the world, there is going to be an emotional connection. They are going to be happy to share.

If you had said something like, "Asia? I've never been there. What was that trip like?" you would have opened up the door for a longer and more real conversation.

Look for those nuggets in small talk that can open women up.

Asking for the Digits

Before you ask, check for these things.

Check for that ring on her left hand. Make sure you didn't miss it. You don't want to realize you are hitting on a married woman. All good?

Did she say she's seeing someone? Some guys think that if she's got a boyfriend, she's still up for some fun. She's not married.

I think this is disrespectful and makes you less of a man. If you had a girlfriend and some guy tried to make a move, how would you react? It's one thing for her to say she has one, but if you know, back off. Treat her the same way you would want your own girlfriend treated.

Assume It's Going to Happen

Be confident that you two are going to go out and have fun. Don't say, "Is it ok if I ask you out?" You don't need permission to ask her. Just ask!

Be specific. Say, "Would you have dinner with me?" or "Maybe let's have dinner." Assume that she's just had a great conversation, and of course, she's going to want to see more of you! Come up with a day as soon as you can.

Snap a Picture

If you are somewhere interesting, offer to snap a photo and text it to her. You'll get her number. If getting her number doesn't seem right at the moment, offer to post it on Instagram and ask what her profile is and follow her. Then tag the photo and contact her online.

Use What You Have Learned

I will bet you that she has provided you with at least a dozen different ways to ask her out, but you didn't even realize it.

As she tells you things about herself, look for the information. What has she said she has wanted to do but never had the chance? You probably aren't in a position to take her to Paris, but if she said she's never had French food, ask her out to a French dinner. Does she want to see the new award-winning dramatic film coming out next week?

Say you should go together.

During your conversation, you are getting to know her, and the truth is she is telling you exactly what to do. She has told you her likes and dislikes, so you just need to figure out the best one for her right then.

Make sure it's one you can do right away. If she says she's excited about a movie coming out in six months, not a good idea to pursue that. You don't want to wait six months for a date. Or if there's a club or restaurant she's interested in but hasn't opened yet, don't wait. Find your opportunities!

Topics to Avoid

- Your Exes

While it is common to find common ground with your past relationships, this can turn negative pretty quickly. Instead of having a positive experience and enjoying each other, you are going to bring up bad memories on both sides. Commiseration is not stimulating conversation that turns people on.

- Personal Trauma

Unless you're talking to this woman at some sort of support group, try to avoid any discussion of past personal trauma until you've known her for a while. (And if you did meet her at such a group, remember to focus on healing first and being part of a support system for your fellow survivors, not getting laid by the cute girl by the snack table.) Trauma can be a real bonding agent, and women want you to be open with them about your feelings—later in the relationship. Even mental health problems, something which we should always try to normalize so that people won't be afraid to seek help, should wait until you two are more comfortable with each other.

Until then, don't use this to propel a conversation, even if she provides you with the perfect opening. You don't want to scare her away.

- TMI

Do you recall a commercial where the woman is on a first date with this guy, and when the guy mentions how awkward first dates can be, she replies, "Yeah, like my constipation"? You would hope that this commercial is just an exaggeration meant for comedic effect, but you'd be surprised. Some people really do share way too much in their first conversation with someone, especially if they get nervous or run out of things to say. Avoid this at all costs.

Obviously, bodily functions are off-limits. So is bragging about your sexual prowess or how hung you are. Like I said before, talk about love and passion, not sex. Besides, those organs are just not something women—or anyone—want to hear about when they first meet you. Gross.

Remember, use innuendo, but be subtle. Don't be TMI.

- Politics and Religion

Eventually, this can become a wealth of conversation, but at first, be very careful bringing up politics and religion until you know where both of you stand.

Don't editorialize or go on about your personal beliefs, especially religion. If you go to church, say so but don't make her think you are highly religious and almost became a priest. If you aren't religious, don't lie and say you are, instead just touch on it, saying you're not that religious. If it gets to the third and fourth date, then start talking about these things. But not yet.

- Sports

She may love sports, but the vast majority of women don't want to talk about it all the time and definitely not the breakdown of box scores or how you can remember the entire line-up of the 2016 World Champion Chicago Cubs baseball team.

She's probably going to ask if you watch sports and which ones. Tell her the truth, but don't dwell on it. She's trying to find out if it's such a dominating thing that it would potentially take away from the time you two might spend together.

Ask her if she watches or enjoys sports. Often women connect sports to emotional events, like family outings to games as a kid or watching football on Sundays with her dad.

You, however, most likely connect it to certain events, like the once-in-a-lifetime comeback you watched or an amazing play or the time a player got injured, and they showed it over and over on replay.

So, find her connection. And never belittle other sports because they aren't the ones you watch. Don't start saying how stupid golf or soccer is because you might just find out she does it every weekend. Even if you have rival teams, don't belittle her for cheering for them. A bit of good-natured teasing is fine, but make sure to keep it in check.

Last Resort

If you don't think anything will work and you don't know what to do…

Just ask her!

Just come right out and ask, no matter what the conversation has been like. You don't have to lead up to it. If you felt like there was a connection, then just ask her.

Sometimes you just need to take a chance.

Chapter 5:

From Small Talk to Deep Conversation

W hen you start talking to a girl, it is best to let the conversation flow naturally and not be too controlling. Non-confrontational interaction is a good way of approaching a girl and allows her to meet you where you are at. It also makes sure that she will not be uncomfortable with your advances. The best way to do this is by being talkative, as this will give people confidence.

It is easier to have a conversation if you are in a group rather than one-on-one. A group gives you more talking partners, and hence if you are not good in conversation, you can just choose to talk to another person as it seems natural. Moreover, when you are part of a group, there is more structure on how the conversation should flow.

When using small talk, the trick is not to make it useful but rather, it just helps us connect with each other. It creates a good first impression, and a conversation that is too heavy can put a person off. In a group, it is better for you to speak in the others' pauses rather than speak under your breath. It gives the impression that you are comfortable enough to start chatting with people you just met. This is also the time to show your confidence as you are relaxed and find out whether she has any interesting friends.

When approaching strangers, do not go straight up to her and start talking about her job and other personal stuff. Use small talk initially and then gradually transition to deeper conversation. You can start by asking about people's names, where they are from, and how everybody met, for example. Let the conversation flow naturally in order for you to get carried away with it.

On the other hand, do not rely on small talk too much as this is just useless banter and may make you come across as a bore. It is also important not to overdo being funny as this will only make the atmosphere awkward. Ideally, you would want to end up in a situation where there are no pauses during your conversation or when speaking with her. You should be careful though, that while you keep her talking, she does not end up answering all questions without your input in a normal conversation. You must also try to make sure that the person or group has enough people in it so that you have someone else to go back and speak with.

A good way of getting into a flow so that the conversation flows easily is by using both small talk and deep conversation during a single conversation. Just before you end your conversation, let the other person go first by commenting on something you did not mention earlier and thank her for the conversation. This will show your appreciation as opposed to just leaving without saying thanks. You should also avoid giving her last-minute surprises such as asking her for your number or not letting them finish their meal without letting them know what you are doing next.

If she is single, you should try to start talking about what you like and how you are looking for a relationship that is right and not just one based on physical attraction. You should also initiate the conversation as opposed to she talking about herself to you first or talking about her preferences in men and how she sees herself. The best way to do this is by asking her questions about what she likes in a man without making it sound obvious. For example, ask whether she prefers someone who embraces her or someone who surprises her.

You should also make sure that the conversation doesn't drag on as much when there are several people present. You should ask questions that keep the conversation going or things that let you help in the situation. You should also avoid asking too many questions as this can be seen as difficult and intrusive. This will make women see you as a person who is interested in her rather than a weirdo who is just trying to get to know her.

Introduce the opposite sex to each other, especially if they are not close friends. Doing this helps you break down any tension that may be caused due to not knowing who would talk and what they would choose to talk about. It also gives you time for your conversation with her, and if this goes well, she could introduce you to some of her friends which you could then meet at a later date.

Keep the topics of conversation to what both of you are comfortable with. For example, if you are not interested in sports and she is, do not talk about it. It is alright if you ask her what she likes or what her interests are. This gives her a hint that you are interested in getting to know her more than just finding out whether she knows anything about football. You will find that when it comes to sports, it is so easy for a girl who likes them to bore you with endless statistics and facts that would repulse any man who does not follow up on football or any other sports they like.

Avoid letting the conversation drop while you are out with a girl unless you have just started talking to her. Some men will be quite interested in her and want to get her number or perhaps take her out, but they just get stuck in a position whereby the conversation is coming to an end and then doing nothing about it.

The best way to understand what the other person is feeling is by keeping an eye on their body language. If she looks warm, it means the conversation is flowing well. But if she breaks the flow by asking you a question or handing you the coat she borrowed from you, then this means that she isn't feeling comfortable with what you are saying.

You should also be careful not to say anything that might make her feel uncomfortable or cause her to feel like she was being judged by you unconsciously. You will, however, find that most girls will show a reaction in situations like these and not just let it slide as it might hurt her feelings. If this happens, you should apologize and try to make her feel better. You should also try to avoid saying things that may be offensive to the girl even if they were not meant as such.

This point is important, especially when you have just met a girl for the first time and have not had time to get to know her very well or she has had no time with you either. Therefore, knowing how she feels through her body language can help you avoid making mistakes later when she becomes more comfortable with you.

When in conversation, both parties must be comfortable with what the other person is saying. This is important as if one person feels uncomfortable with how the conversation is going or what the conversation partner is saying, it can make the other person feel uncomfortable too.

It is important when having a conversation that both parties are listening actively and not just waiting for their turn to talk again. This is because when she is talking, she is not only trying to give you a message but also trying to see if you are paying attention to what she is saying. Therefore, when she feels that you are not paying attention, she may get distracted from the conversation, and as a result, an uncomfortable situation may arise between the two of you. Hence it is important that you listen actively by asking questions or making comments throughout the whole conversation so that she can feel engaged instead of just feeling like she has to talk all the time. You should also try to avoid too many interruptions while speaking, especially when it doesn't seem necessary and just for your own benefit, mainly so that the conversation can flow properly.

Chapter 6:

Texting Tips to Get More Dates

A lot of guys do text girls but come out sloppy and sometimes purposeless. A man just takes the number and starts circumventing and going round in circles until he becomes notoriously a bother. Some men also have aims for texting, yet they cannot get them across through the text. Aimless texts that do not seem to be tied to a purpose do not elicit emotion or grip the girl with a sense of awe.

You should know that a man can only have two objectives to text a girl, that is noted as the sister, business partner, or client; to either establish friendship through the building of rapport or to get the girl to agree to a date. However, the core aim and the paramount one is that you should be able to get the girl to meet up with you. There are guys who come out with a maligned objective of just hanging around with endless texting and hop back and forth to a fortunate date with her. This is quite timid, redundant, and could veer into the quarters of irritation to the girl.

When you do not have an objective, the girl starts to wonder if you do not have someone else to tell the sort of things you are texting her with. The girl wants you to come out focused and sharp, ensuring you that nothing gets messy. Do not let your target get lost in the process of engaging in chit-chat. So that means that do not mix up texting her to establish a relationship base, perhaps as a precursor to friendship and texting her to just secure a date. If you want to meet her, you want to meet her and focus on making that happen.

Avoid circumventing around your goal as you will confuse yourself. You will find yourself sending too many texts to which no replies will be forthcoming. Come out bold and courageous. Appear sure and exude confidence that that is what you are, and it gets you the results you want. Having known the objective of texting, then you can focus on the matter in the texts.

Text Warm and Cold

There are two forms of texting in light of the objectives stated above. Cold-texting and Warm-Texting. When you text a girl that has an anticipative mindset and is minding you at the moment you text her, that is warm texting. Cold texting is when the girl is probably oblivious to you and has no expectation that you are going to text her.

This distinction is important since you are supposed to know how far you are going to get the girl from in order to be able to put everything set towards attaining your objective on her. You are supposed to tune the way the texts come out to match her level of readiness for you.

Texting A Girl to Drive Towards A Date

When you want to build rapport first, it may take some schedule that can be quite rigorous. Start by texting her for several days to build a base of mutual interest, perhaps. After you have met her and she shares her contact with you, initiate communication through text and invite her to some engagement for the sake of socializing or mingling. You will, therefore, need to keep the conversation following the approaches of keeping a conversation going. However, do not take it into over a week before you are already at the point of arranging for a meet-up. So typically, you will be texting her with a date slated to come in a few days, maybe five days away.

But better for you if you could not engage in rapport building. This is unless you perceive the girl to be one that requires you to take her through such an adventure. When you have secured the number, proceed to your main goal already without heeding the urge of trying to win her. This requires you to stop selling yourself as a brand like you are an item. The point just goes straight to making the girl go out with you. Obviously, rapport building will fall into place by itself.

You should first come out warm and with charm in your texts. This is in order for you to lower the girl's defenses and avoid alerting her to be suspicious and resistant. Then ensure that you have something of value that you appear to be offering. Whatever that is could be imagined or illusionary, but it should be able to get the girl drooling with curiosity. It could also simply the fun thing that she desires to be doing, which is to meet you. Only that she is laying back to let you lead her there. So, a girl will text some messages that may be destructive such as, "How is your day going?" Answer but ensure that she does not get you entangled into sideshows that sidetrack you. Keep steering towards your goal regardless of what you are talking about.

The text thread could appear like this;

Man: Lisa, hello! I am thinking we could work on creating time to get some snacks. Could this weekend be appropriate for you?

Girl: The weekend is usually free apart from my routine to spring clean the house. What is for dinner?

Man: arranging to cook. So, you could do the cleaning and then you are free. It sounds workable for me. We do this at 3 pm. I know you are going to like it at the Pop Club.

Girl: Looks hurried, but will set me for it.

Man: I look forward to it, see you on Saturday.

See how the meet-up comes through quite fast and ready. It only had to take being focused on the goal. When she asked about dinner, the guy does not switch subject to discussing food and how it is going to be cooked or what is going to be cooked. You may risk being supped out of all seductive energy when she entangles you in questioning or succeeds in getting you to overexpose yourself to her, which makes her judge you. Push your agenda and appear clinical as opposed to being blunt and unfocused.

A strategy could be to use the first meeting to suggest that you could get out a bit before you even take her number. This is something that can make the process a lot easier than waiting to pursue a date fresh on text. The good thing here is that asking for the date first before getting physical with her makes the girl have more readiness for you. It just even makes your next move of asking for her number easier as that is the only way that the date will get set up.

You have an opportunity to ask the girl to go out with you in person, and you should not squander it. Do not wait for the text-only, as perhaps she could think you are not confident enough to just get out and get what you want. So, seize the moment to get things started on an auspicious note. For instance, when you are conversing, in person, with her and she is explaining something, you steer it to your aim;

Girl: (in the course of a conversation at the place you have met) …. I had to really get out of the place and save her from an awkward moment. She was almost freaking out.

Man: Haaa, you mean? That was so intuitive of you.

Girl: we girls feel nervous when awkward moments happen, so I just had to be a great friend.

Man: and on that note, I think we are going to go back to the club; your fun was cut short when you left. How is your weekend looking?

Girl: well, that will depend. I will need to confirm.

Man: That is fine, so what is your number? I will text you.

Girl: 5672….

How hard was that? You are immediately working on your objective at the first meeting, and the texting only comes later as a follow-up. She will now not be surprised when you text her, and you are not concerned about rapport building but rather remind her to confirm her availability for the Sunday date. This can help you seduce a girl in the way that you expend lesser efforts yet get back huge rewards. In fact, going y this, I could demand you to right away go into your contacts to delete all of the numbers of girls you took and whom you did not suggest to go out with at the first meeting.

Icebreaker Text

Also, focus on ensuring you are good at breaking the ice by avoiding taking too long before you can text the girl. The longer you hesitate or "dilly dally" in sending the text, the weirder it will just get for you. She keeps wondering if you will send her a text at all or simply moves on and forgets having met and exchanged contacts with you. You also start to pile up thoughts in your head as you overthink that will naturally make you come out rather awkward.

The way out is to execute the icebreaker. This will immediately set you free as your fear of how the conversation will go has been dispatched. Having sent the icebreaker text, it imparts into the girl some sense of anticipation that you will probably text her further in the coming moments. It will also help you that when you eventually text her for a cat, you will not have the need to start saying who you are, and hence you have a head start in getting busy to pursue your objective. An example of a text to break the ice is;

Man: I just had a great time with you in the lobby. I did not notice the time pass. Nice hooking up, your latest friend :) Hudson

Or

Man: It has been an exciting time talking to you. Steve here.

You could keep it as short as possible just to ensure she does not already get thinking she has taken your breath away. You are being careful to also not appear needy and desperate. The icebreaker will appear quite infectious yet portray you as one who is used to meeting new girls, and it is not quite much of a big deal. You are also using a friend to tease her a bit and get her attention. She will be pondering if you mean to be interested or if you are neutral towards her. She hopes you come out to clear this confusion. However, if you sense that the girl is already on your radar and likes you already, avoid using "friend." This is for the girl who is flattered that you gave her attention and that you have class over her. Do not use "friend" to make her feel snubbed or despair that she can't have you.

59

Chapter 7:

Examples of Text Conversations

Men call women who give them their phone numbers but avoid meeting them in person are flakes. Numerous men's forums on the internet are dedicated to flakes and how to prevent flaking. Given our problem-solving nature, it is not surprising that we men have come up with a variety of ways to account for the impact of flakes on our love lives. Some men schedule dates with two or more women at the same time to account for the possibility of one of the women flaking on him. Others use a variety of ethically worrisome texting tactics to coerce women into not being flakes. While I applaud these men for their ingenuity and fighting spirit, I think they missed the boat by not addressing the crux of the problem.

Women flake on men because men fail to demonstrate their high sexual market value during texting exchanges with them. If these men were strategic about using their texts to playfully and effectively communicate to these women the fact that they are masculine men who have high social status and are preselected by women, women would not flake on them. In fact, ever since I figured out how to emphasize these attributes about myself in my communications with women, no woman has flaked on me.

Use text messages to subtly communicate your high sexual market value.

Thus, you must subtly imply that you are a high-status man instead of explicitly stating it in your text messages. Being terse, gently, and playfully disqualifying her statements, making her wait for your responses to her text messages for at least as long as she makes you wait for her responses to your text messages, giving her directives, and occasionally providing approval help create this implication in her mind.

Also, you must implicitly suggest that you have other sexual options instead of explicitly stating it. A great method to accomplish this is by demonstrating that you are indifferent to getting her approval and not concerned about her losing interest in you. Indifference can be shown in a variety of ways, such as using poor grammar and punctuation, ignoring her questions, teasing her playfully, and responding without emotion to her actions.

Exercise caution when texting women to avoid triggering their auto-rejection mechanisms

Demonstrating a high sexual market value via texting requires one to be cautious as well. If a woman feels that you are too good for her, she will suspect that one or more of the following statements is true and try to confirm her suspicions:

- You want to pump and dump her.
- You will be an unfaithful boyfriend.
- Your interest in her is not genuine, and you have ulterior motives.
- You are actually not as great as she thinks you are.

In her mind, the following question is of paramount importance –

why would such an attractive man, who can be with women who are more attractive than me, be so interested in me? The longer this question remains unanswered in her mind, the more likely a woman is to auto-reject you when you fail to escalate your interaction with her to the next level. When she auto-rejects you, she will take any of your minor flaws and blow them up out of proportion to convince herself that you are not good enough for her. The more insecure a woman is about her appearance, the more often this emotional self-defense mechanism rears its ugly head.

To avoid being auto-rejected by a woman during texting interactions with her, you must never explicitly say anything negative to her in your text messages. Needless to say, any sort of teasing or flirting must be done very playfully. If you need to punish her bad behavior, you can ignore her texts and not respond to them for a pre-determined period of time, make your texts terser and/or cryptic, or respond to her texts very erratically.

Avoiding auto-rejection will be especially important for you if you are an attractive man because you can trigger a woman's auto-rejection mechanism by simply making a few jokes at her expense. Let us look at a very detailed example of a text message-based conversation in which I subtly communicated my high sexual market value to a woman without triggering her auto-rejection mechanism. My comments are italicized.

S: I learned how to boil water last year, and I'm pretty proud of it! Far from sashimi, but hey, I'm trying lol 3:42 PM

A day later

Me: I bet YOU don't even need to turn the gas on for that. 3:47 PM

I responded a day later, showing I was unafraid of her losing interest in me. Also, I teased her, implying that I have high social status.

S: Sure don't! Just bought an electric kettle. 3:48 PM

Me: Well, played 3:48 PM

I gave her my approval, implying that I have high social status.

S: How was ur weekend? Go on crazy dates again? 3:49 PM

Me: No crazy ones, missed a flight to the Dominican Republic, ended up chilling in Vienna 4:02 PM

I made her wait for my response, implying that I have high social status. Also, I implied that I did go on dates with other women.

S: What?! How the heck did that happen? Oooh, I'd be pissed. Have u been before? 4:14 PM

S: Did the possessive one try to see u again? I'd be like, sorry I'd rather watch paint dry...at least that's my excuse lol 4:15 PM

Me: friend-zoned her, what happened w your nice date? 4:33 PM

I ignored her first question to show my indifference to her walking away. I made her wait for 18 minutes to Pooh show my indifference to her walking away from this conversation. Also, by admitting to friend-zoning a girl for being too possessive, I implied that I have many sexual options.

Me: Shit happens. I fly every week 4:35 PM

I gave a very vague and brief answer to imply that I have high social status.

63

S: Nice date offered to make dinner last week, but a killer migraine made an appearance, so I canceled. Yikes, I hear ya. Hope u got airline credit. What do 4:41 PM

S: u do that has u flying every week? 4:41 PM

Me: Wow, that's a lot of effort on his part 4:53 PM

I made her wait for my response and ignored her question to show my indifference to her walking away from this conversation. Also, I subtly passed judgment on her date to imply that I have high social status.

S: He's def nice but not feeling a spark. Could be bc this is my first crack at dating since the last guy. Boohoo 5:04 PM

S: I even wore a sexy black dress. 5:05 PM

She sends a picture for me to see.

Me: U have a very mischievous grin 5:20 PM

I complimented her but not about her dress to avoid qualifying to her. Also, I made her wait for my response for 15 minutes to imply that I have high social status.

S: I disagree! Ur mancandy in a suit 5:26 PM

Me: Wow. 5:32 PM

She made me wait for 6 minutes, so I made her wait for 6 minutes. Also, I didn't act all that excited about receiving a compliment from her to show my indifference to getting her approval.

S: Yes. A compliment has been earned...don't get used to it!!! 5:36 PM

Me: I'm printing your text and putting it on my refrigerator. 5:37 PM

I playfully tease her to keep things light and fun.

S: Oh hell no. Not ok! So, when do we get to meet? Something basic like Starbucks...not asking to roll out the red carpet 6:08 PM

Me: out of town M-thurs, next wknd or quick drink tonight? 6:15 PM

Once again, I make her wait for my response to imply my high social status. Also, my response is in line with my being a high-status man who is never too available.

S: I'll be back in the area around 8:30 today...is 9 too late for you? If so, next wknd is totally fine. No rush 6:19 PM

Me: 9 should be fine 6:25 PM

S: Sounds good. Know of a place open past 10? Not looking for a late-night but also don't want to be rushed 6:40 PM

Me: I'll find one. 6:45 PM

S: Cool. Around Vienna/Fairfax is preferred 6:46 PM

Me: I was gonna find a place in SE DC, but ok Vienna/Fairfax it is. 6:47 PM

I take control of the situation like a high-status man while keeping things fun.

S: Lol, you're silly. I'm looking as well. 6:49 PM

Me: Gordon Biersch Brewery at Tyson's corner open till 11, see you at 9 7:28 PM

I don't reply back for about 50 minutes to avoid seeming needy. And, by expecting her to follow my lead, I imply my high social status.

S: Sounds good! 7:32 PM

S: Ok to meet at 9:15? Bus from NY had a slight delay 7:58 PM

Me: K 8:50 PM

I do not respond to her text for about an hour to imply that something or someone more important than her is keeping me busy.

We meet for drinks. She texts me about five minutes after our date ended.

S: Glad we got a chance to meet up! Really enjoyed talking to you. Drive safely, safe travels this week, and get some sleep tonight! 12:22 AM

Me: I had fun too. Just got home. Gnite 12:26 AM

I give no indication of my future plans and use terse wording to imply I might have other, more attractive options.

Chapter 8:
Dos and Don'ts in Texting

Here are guidelines to assist you to up your texting game effortlessly.

DO Text a Girl Quickly

I don't understand guys that see a text from a girl and wait 30 minutes or an hour to reply. If you see a text, reply to it. There is no point analyzing the time it took the girl to text you back so you can take longer to reply. If the girl starts to see a pattern and realize what you are doing, she will discover what an immature, needy guy you are and be instantly turned off.

Dating is about creating connections with one another, having fun, and being flirty with another person. It's not about studying the time it took for the other person to reply.

One of the major downfalls of the "pick-up" and dating community is things overcomplicated for no reason.

It's simple. If you see a text from a girl, you reply to it.

If both of you are replying quickly to each other, you are more likely to have a fun conversation that flows. You will build momentum, which is crucial for when you are ready to ask her on a date.

Remember how we talked about texting her to create emotions? Well, how are you supposed to create emotions if you are texting each other hours apart?

But What If the Girl Is Taking Forever to Reply?

Before you start texting girls, get a life. There will be times where you take a while to reply too, since you have an awesome life.

The girl will notice that you have a life, and your world doesn't revolve around her, which shows independence and self-confidence. It will make her much more attracted to you.

DO Text Her Enough to Get Her Interested

I see many guys try to text as little as possible to show that they are "hard to get." When you start texting a girl you just met, it is natural for you to put more effort than her. You are trying to "prove" that you are a cool guy.

The girl won't be receptive to you straight away because her defense mechanism is up. When girls meet a new guy for the first time, they have this imaginary little shield to protect them. This shield goes up because you are a stranger to the girl. She doesn't know you, which means she doesn't trust you. If she doesn't trust you, she won't flirt with you or show you her true personality.

What you need to do is put effort into your texts to show her that you are a cool, laid-back, light-hearted guy, so her imaginary little shield gets lowered. Once the shield is lowered, that's when she starts letting her personality shine through. That's when she starts flirting back.

Give it time at the start and put in some effort. The girl won't fall in love with you overnight. You need to text the girl just enough to get her interested and build momentum to get her to start thinking about you.

DON'T Use Cheesy Emoji's

There are only two emojis you should use—either the flirty one or the laughing one. All other emojis are pointless.

These are the two most masculine emojis available. Please don't use the monkey faces or kissing emojis. These just make you seem more feminine. If someone was to read your texting conversations and think you are a girl, then you need to ease up on the emojis.

This brings me on to my next point...

DO Use Emoji's Sparingly

The only time you should use emojis is when you are trying to show your true intentions. If you are teasing the girl, then adding a laughing emoji will let her know you are just kidding around.

Do use the laughing emojis sparingly. Don't spam the girl with 7 laughing faces with every reply you send. One is enough, maybe two if what she said was funny. If you start to overuse the laughing face, you won't seem genuine, and it will turn the girl off.

Lastly, please don't use "Haha" or "Lol." You have emoji's available to you; use them.

If you are unsure whether you should use an emoji or not... don't. You can overuse emojis, but you can't underuse them.

DO Tease Her

You should always tease a girl. It shows her that you're not a suck-up and that you don't put her on a pedestal.

Teasing also creates fun, flirty conversations, which is exactly what you want to be doing. You can always use the laughing emoji to show that you are teasing her and that you're not being serious.

Many times I have been in conversation with girls where I would tease them and forget to put a laughing emoji resulting in them thinking I was being serious. The laughing emoji is a lifesaver; use it wisely.

DON'T Text Her All Day

No matter how awesome your life is, you should never text the girl all day, every day, unless the girl is doing the same. I say this because you need to invest just as much as the girl does for a real connection to be created.

Don't text her all day if she isn't doing the same. The girl doesn't want to know every single little detail about your life. It makes you seem desperate. If you're texting her all day, then you are telling her you don't have an interesting life, and your whole world revolves around her.

There is no way you are texting other girls or having a good life if you are texting her 24/7. You should provide her some space to invest; let her miss you a bit. If she knows that every time she turns her Wi-Fi on, or she looks at her phone, she will have a message from you, then that takes the excitement out of texting. You want girls to be eagerly checking their phones, wondering if you have texted them or not yet.

If it helps you, put your phone on silent for an hour while you do something that makes you happy, or work on something that adds value to your life.

I hate it when I'm spending time with my best friend, and every time we start a conversation, we are forced to stop the conversation every two minutes so he can text a girl. Not only does it make him seem more invested in the girl, but it's also annoying because we can't have a real face-to-face conversation with no interruption.

DON'T Always Text Her First

If you're constantly texting first, it shows that you are more into her than she is into you. No matter what you say, if a girl never, if not rarely, texts first, then she just isn't that much into you. I don't care how shy or nervous she is; after a few fun interactions with you, she will text you first if she wants you that badly.

A great way to determine if a girl is into you is to not text her. I realize this statement contradicts the purpose of this book but trust me. After you have been texting back and forth for some time and are having fun, flirty conversation…stop texting her. Don't text her for a few days. If she texts you, that means she is into you. If not, then she might not be as into you as you thought. Always run this test after you create some initial attraction.

Also, no good morning texts. Leave this for when you are in a relationship. Good morning text show that you are way more invested in her than she is in you. It shows that you think about her not only before you go to sleep but right after you wake up.

She is going to think your whole world revolves around her.

DON'T Talk Too Much

Most guys are always trying to think hard for the perfect message to send the girl. Perfection doesn't exist. The same goes for texting.

If you can't think of what to say and see that the conversation is dying down...let it. There is no need for you to keep trying to revive the conversation when you can see that it's not going anywhere.

By not saying anything, you give the girl some space to invest too. If you think it's a good time to end the conversation, end it. Don't be afraid to let go.

DO Use Text to Set Up a Date

The whole purpose of texting is to set up a date with a girl. It is not getting to know her or trying to get nudes from her. It's to get her to go out with you so you can have a face-to-face interaction.

You should always set up dates through text and not through the phone for one simple reason. It is so much easier for the girl to say yes through text than it is through the phone. If you haven't even properly met the girl yet, a phone call will be a bit awkward and might scare her off. Stick with texting.

When you set up a date through text, you should never ASK a girl to go out on a date. Forget about "Being a gentleman." You must make it seem like a mutual decision.

You need to be the dominant male and ask a girl to JOIN you or make the assumption that she wants to see you. When you ASK the girl out, it subconsciously sounds like the date is going to be boring or awkward.

For example, don't say, "Hey, you want to go out on a date with me Saturday night?" or "Can I take you out Saturday night?". Instead, say, "Hey, you're pretty cool; we should hang out. I'm free Saturday night, you down?".

This shows dominance and the fact that it subconsciously sounds like you are going to have a good time.

Chapter 9:
Using Social Media

D ating is hard. Aside from getting her to go on a date with you, the other way to get a girl interested in you is by initiating conversations and using your social media skills to build rapport.

Here, we'll talk about different ways of building rapport that doesn't suck and possibly even develops an attraction. This also includes what social media platforms are the best for connection building, as well as how you can use them most efficiently.

What is Social Media?

Let's talk about what social media is. Basically, it's a platform that connects individuals through technology. For example, Facebook connects people through a network where users can share content, communicate with others and get updates on their friends' lives and activities. Twitter has a similar system, but it uses hashtags and short messages (140 characters or less).

On Instagram, there are no words or actual conversations. It's a way to present yourself visually to the world and share your day-to-day experiences by taking photos that are aesthetically pleasing in both form and content.

Nowadays, there are numerous social media platforms such as Pinterest, Tumblr, Snapchat, etc. But the four we've mentioned are the most popular and widely used, along with dating apps like Tinder.

But why spend time on social media at all? After all, if you're trying to get a girl's number so that you can further things in the real world, why not just meet her in person? Is there any reason to invest time on social media?

The truth is: Social media is an excellent way to get a girl's attention for online dating or even to initiate contact with her if she's already your friend. Social media allows you to meet women without having to leave the house. All you need is a strong profile, a good-looking photo, and well-written posts.

Benefits of Social Media

The benefits of having a social media presence are vast, to say the least:

- It allows you to connect with girls you like directly without having to go through intermediaries (like mutual friends).
- It provides you the opportunity to display your personality to the world and show off your identity – both of which are excellent for attracting girls.
- It can help build rapport with girls that may not have been possible under normal circumstances. After all, it is a way to connect with them virtually. Even if you didn't know each other previously, social media could allow you to become friends or even start dating.
- It can give you an extra edge should you be communicating with a girl whom you want to meet in real life. It might even serve as proof that you actually like her. For example, if you're trying to convince her that she's wrong about something and she sees how assertive/friendly you are on social media

through photos, this could win her over and make her more amenable to meeting up in the real world for a date.

Get Started Today

I know it's hard, but it will pay off in the long run.

The idea is simple: You start your profile and post some photos of yourself so that girls will know who they're talking to when they see your profile name or name tag.

You also create a strong and attractive profile picture, preferably one that is as visually appealing as possible. Take your profile as a business card. You want her to see that you're handsome, confident, smart, interesting, and confident. You must really believe in yourself so that she will too.

When you post your first update/photo, be sure to make yourself sound interesting enough so that she'll want to know more about you. This means talking about something or sharing something interesting with her that applies to either you or the group she's in (community) so that it's not just random chat talk. For example, if your friend is in the army, a photo of military vehicles or soldiers could work.

You can also talk about experiences in your life or things that you did recently. You don't have to be boring or over-talkative though. Just make sure your updates are relevant to what you're writing and what she's about so that she feels like she really knows you.

You should also link her profile with yours so that she can follow/find you and vice versa. This will ensure that when they see each other in person, they know where each other are coming from and what "type of people" they'll be dealing with.

Finally, make sure your updates are unique and interesting without being over-the-top or too provocative.

Once you get the hang of things, you can start making connections with girls, building rapport, and possibly deepening it into a relationship. Also, remember that these methods are great for developing attraction in women, so you're on the right track if they seem to be liking what they see.

You won't know when you've succeeded until they send you a message, tell you something about themselves, or even ask you out on a date.

Hows

<u>How to know if she's using this too and how to make your social media presence interesting to women</u>

At first, some people just want to see what's the big deal about social media. They don't have any interest in meeting up in real life or convincing anyone that they're interested in them; they just want to see what all the hype is about and how it can help them meet guys.

The problem with this is that there really isn't much of a secret social media "goldmine" for guys at the moment.

The only real way you can tell if a girl uses social media to find guys is to look at their profile. If you notice that she's too much of a premium user (e.g., has a lot of likes, follows, or fans), then it's very likely that she's using this method to try and "game" guys for dates, relationships, or even sex – which is something that needs to be avoided.

On the other hand, if you see that she has too little of these kinds of things going on, then it's not much of an indicator either way (because this could just mean the above point).

The only way you can really tell is to find out more about her and see if she seems open to the idea of meeting up in the real world or expressing interest in you. If not, then just move on.

If you're interested in making your social media presence interesting to women, then make sure that your updates reflect your personality and that they are funny while still being intriguing (not too provocative or sexual) so that they're worth checking out when the girls see them. The same goes for photos. If you're using photos of other people (like friends),m then make sure that they'll attract a girl's attention enough for them to want to check you out for themselves.

How to know if she wants to meet up in real life (make a date)

If you follow the above advice and make yourself interesting on social media, then you'll have the opportunity to ask a girl out on a date. Whether or not she accepts is another thing, but at least you've tried. It's also likely that if she's interested in meeting up with guys, then she will be open to talking about it with you.

Some of these indicators can be obvious – i.e., her commenting on your picture or video, liking it, and then sending you a message. If she does this, then it lends itself to an easy transition into an actual conversation about meeting up in person (via text message or social media).

Similarly, if she's commenting on your posts on her wall, her friends' walls, and making comments that are similar to the way she would comment on your photo/video if she wanted to meet up – then this is also a good sign.

Then there are the not-so-obvious signs like her inviting you to events that she's going to or ones that you can both go to. If she's really into meeting up with other guys, then she'll make it as much about you finding someone as it is about her finding someone. She'll be more than happy to set you up with another female friend of hers and so on and so forth.

Yes, this might, on some occasions, feel like she's just being nice, but even if that's the case – it still means that there's a decent chance that you'll be able to meet up with her in person at some point in the future.

It might also mean that you're being set up in a platonic way for someone else who would like to meet you too. After all, most people don't want to be set up with their friends' ex-girlfriends, and so it's a very nice way for someone else to let you know about them. It's just polite, really.

What Social Media Platforms to Use

1. Facebook

Facebook is one of the social media platforms famous for attracting women and initiating conversation with them. It has a very user-friendly interface, which makes it ideal for anyone interested in using its features.

You can use Facebook to meet new people or reconnect with old friends as well (and this last point is something that you should keep in mind). If you're already using Facebook to connect with your female friends, then great. If not, then you better start now!

All you need is a profile picture (preferably showing only your face) and a strong title (that's also eye-catching). These are the two things that people tend to look at first when they see your profile name or name tag, and so it's important that they work for you.

You can also post updates that will attract attention from other users based on the posts you make. Be sure to do this in a fun way as well so that she thinks she's getting some good entertainment value out of your updates.

You'll be able to connect with other girls on Facebook easily – just like the rest of the world does – but try not to overdo it with people who don't really give a damn about you. This is just common courtesy and shows that you're not materialistic.

If you want to make things easier, you can also create an entirely unconnected profile on Facebook and then start using it for updates, photos and posts only once you get more comfortable with the platform.

Another thing you can do is add her to your existing company's Facebook account. This will help you to connect with her seamlessly and will allow her to see all your updates when she goes online through that account.

You can also use Facebook as a platform for teasing girls that you're interested in because there are many memes, jokes, and articles about how good it is to keep a girl waiting (for example, have them wait for your approval before they talk with them). If a girl likes the fact that other girls are on there waiting for you to come online and approve them, then she'll be more likely to talk with you.

2. Twitter

Twitter is another platform that will help you connect with plenty of people from all over the world. It's also extremely visual, so you can actually show off photos and videos that you post. It is likewise a great platform you can use to impress people because it has very little text, and much emphasis is put on images.

It can be a very fun way of communicating with girls too, especially if they're interested in meeting up in real life with some guys (although this doesn't work for everyone). If you're using it to connect with girls, then you'll be able to follow them without them knowing, and they'll see that you're following them (as long as your account isn't private).

Just like on Facebook, you can also use Twitter as a platform for teasing girls too – if they're into it of course! For example, send out tweets that will cause them to react:

I love your shirt. 3 day notice? #tuesday

I just got back to work from vacation wearing the same underwear I packed 3 years ago. #tuesday

I'm having a sleepover with the weatherman. Wish me luck. #tuesday

3. Instagram

Instagram is another visual platform that has a lot of users around the world. It's also very flexible too because it allows you to post all kinds of photos, and not just pictures: video, short clips, memes, quotes, and anything else you can think of. It's also easy to share photos and videos from other social media sites like Facebook so that you don't have to take them from your phone.

Instagram is probably the most popular social media site for guys to use when it comes to attracting women because of how beautiful and appealing it can be when used correctly. It's a great way of showing girls that you're stylish, like fashion, and also have good taste when it comes to girls (as well as yourself).

If you're using Instagram to connect with other girls, then you'll be able to follow them without having to tweet them first or even see their profile photos. You can also comment on all their photos, essentially commenting on them in a Facebook-like manner: by liking, commenting, or sharing one photo.

You can also choose a female profile to follow so that you get updates from her without having to search for them. If you're interested in making your Instagram account interesting for girls, then be sure to use it in a way as this above piece of advice suggests:

Like and comment on other girls' photos on Instagram. The more likes and comments, the more she'll want to check you out

4. Pinterest and Tumblr

When used correctly, these two social media sites can be very interesting platforms for attracting girls (provided that you're not being creepy or sexual). They're also visually engaging because they allow you to pin images that will draw her attention.

You can pin images of whatever you want to. You can make your Pinterest account interesting for girls by doing the following:

- Post inspirational quotes

- Post funny memes (there are a lot of these on the internet)
- Make collages of photos and pin them (you can even ask her if she likes specific pictures to put in) or put together an album with your favorite pictures of her and screenshots of conversation you've had with her. Don't forget to start a Pinterest board just for this! This is one helluva way to keep that connection going and make her want to see more.
- Pin cute animal pictures too – it doesn't matter whether they're kittens or dogs, etc. Be as creative as you want!

5. Snapchat

Snapchat is a social media platform for sending messages and photos to other people with the press of a button. You send the photos and videos as they're being taken, which means that the girls won't even know when they've been sent. It's kind of like an INSTANT message that doesn't count for anything. This might not be the best social media platform to use if you want to be noticed by girls because it doesn't provide them with any feedback regarding what happened when the messages are being sent (as opposed to other platforms).

You can post photos and videos that will be available to her in real-time. This is a great way to tease girls because they'll think that you're updating them on something, but they won't know what.

You can also use Snapchat to send the girls links to articles or funny pages on the internet. In fact, it's probably easier to do this on Snapchat than anywhere else because you don't even need her number (although it's helpful if you already have it). You just send the Snap, and then she has 30 seconds to view it before it disappears from her screen. If this sounds interesting, then have some fun and get right into it!

Chapter 10:
Handling the First Call

Many guys who get a number from a girl will only spend their time talking with the girl using text. While this is a way to go, if you really want to stand out, you need to make a call to the girl as well. It is going to take some confidence in order to make this call rather than hiding behind some texts. It is also a big risk to giving instance responses rather than getting some time to think about what you would like to say. Most men are going to be worried about what they should say and how do they make the conversation last rather than let it go flat. Follow some of these tips for that first phone call so it can go off without a hitch, and you can get that date.

The Pre-Call:

Before you start calling the girl, you should make sure that your game is on. Sometimes practicing out the things that you want to say before you call the girl, or at least having some sort of list present, can help you get this done easier without as many worries. Write some of these things down, and then have a practice conversation a few times before you call. This can really help if you have the jitters about talking to her and can keep you from slipping up as much during the conversation. Of course the conversation is not going to go exactly the way that you practiced it, but at least you have a little practice and are able to feel a bit more confident before starting.

Work On Your Voicemail

In some cases, the girl may give you a call first. If this does happen, you want to make sure that she will be interested in leaving you a voicemail. Have the message on your voicemail be funny or cute or even leave a little brain teaser. This allows you to have something to talk about when you give her a callback, which will avoid some of the awkward pauses that often come with the phone conversation.

When You Should Call

It is a good idea to call her at some point, but you will also want to make sure that she is available and that you will not be bugging her, and you want to be able to ask her out on a date with plenty of time for preparations, so it does not sound like it was planned last minute. Some of the things that you can keep in mind when you are looking to call a girl include:

Right after getting the phone number—it is sometimes a good idea to call a girl right after you have gotten her number. This helps you to stay in her mind a bit longer, and you can just start it out with making sure that you got the right number. If possible, start the conversation where you left off when you last met to keep things interesting.

Sunday to Wednesday—the best time to call is in between these days. The rest of the days are the ones when people are the busiest, and she will probably be out doing something else. You are going to seem a little pathetic if you are calling and wanting to talk for a long time on a Saturday night. You should also call earlier in the week if you are planning on asking her out so that she has plenty of time to have a clear schedule and can come out with you.

Send a text ahead of time—text the girl before you decide to call her to see if she is busy or available to talk for a while. This allows you to know that she is free and that you will not be bothering her as much as you would just calling on the fly. Of course, another fun thing to do is wait for her to text you because you will then automatically know that she is free and you will not be bothering her. When you receive that text, reply back that you are going to call her in a few seconds. Wait a minute or two and then call. Then she is expecting you to call, and you can get right into the conversation.

Set up your time early—you can even set up the time that you would like to call her as you are getting her number. You can tell her that you would be free on Monday night at 7 pm and see if that time will work for her. This allows you to have free time to call and can get rid of the anxiousness you might be feeling about her not answering the phone at all.

Ready For The Call

It is fine to be a bit nervous during this part of the process, but do not let the rings on the other end scare you. Some men might pick up the phone, but they are so nervous that they hope it will go straight to voicemail so that they do not have to talk to the woman. Take a big breath while you are calling, and start thinking more positively.

When it is the first time that you are calling, it is not a good idea to hang up the phone until it is done. This means that you either need to have a conversation with the girl, or you need to leave a voicemail. Hopefully, you are able to get in touch with the girl so that you can have a conversation and get to know each other, but at least with a voicemail, you are providing an incentive for her to get back to you.

If you do end up leaving a voicemail, make sure that you are doing it in the right way in order to entice her to give you a callback. You can leave almost anything that you would like ranging from a question you would like her to answer, saying something that is kind of crazy, or just mention your last conversation to pique her interest. You can also make the conversation sweet and to the point. Just make sure that you are not just asking her to call you back when she has the time. This does not put a limit on when she can call you, and it could take a week or could be when you are at work, and the phone tag will begin. If you have a certain time that would work best for you, tell her to make things easier.

In some cases, the woman might not be able to call you back for a few days. She might have something going on or might not have realized that there was a message for her. If you do not get a callback, you should wait a few days before trying to call her again.

She Picks It Up

In some cases, the woman is going to actually pick up the phone when you call her. Do not take this as a bad sign. It was exactly what you wanted. But if she does pick up, make sure that you have something to say. You do not want to make the conversation awkward or end up hanging up the phone on her. This goes back to having a few ideas ready and written down, so even if you get stuck, you can help yourself out. You also need to make sure that you are able to keep the conversation going for a while; no one wants to just have a conversation that is a question and then a few word answer. Try to talk about something that interests you as well as her or imagine that you are talking to one of your good friends. The woman will respond in kind, and then the conversation will keep going for a long period of time. Of course, you also need to make a good way to end the conversation since it is not going to go on forever. You could say that you have something going on that you need to go do or even set up the date to end out the call.

As you can see, the phone call with the girl does not have to be as scary as you think. She is as worried about how this will go as you are, so just take a deep breath and have some fun. It does not have to be tedious and can even be an extension of the foundation you have worked on with the texting. Plus, it is going to put you in a much better light with this woman, which can make the whole date go so much better.

Conclusion

Having good phone skills is important because it will facilitate and increase the chances of her meeting you for a date after the initial interaction. Your phone skills are important, but they pale in significance compared with the most important thing, and that is to become a more attractive guy in general.

When you are that guy, your phone game won't even matter that much because the girl will want to see you again. Having said that, here are some important things to remember about phone skills.

Girls give out their numbers all the time. Don't take the act of her giving you her number as any guarantee. It doesn't mean much and is only just a potential at this stage.

Just like girls give out their number a lot, they also flake a lot. Her flaking can be because she was not attracted to you enough or for a multitude of other reasons that are beyond your control. Don't over-analyze the scenario as to why it happened.

The only thing you should be focused on is whether you yourself were attractive enough when you met her and how you will be with the next girl.

When you get her number, text her your name right away or shortly after. She'll know who you are when you text her next. Then over the next few days, send her ping texts that show a playful side to you and keep you on her radar. Avoid texts that convey desperation and that you really want to meet her.

Show her that you're not rushing for the date. Demonstrate abundance and non-neediness. Find the balance between showing enough interest but not making her the most important thing that has happened to you recently.

After a few days of texting here and there, suggest a meet-up. Also, stick to texts instead of calling. Calling runs more risk that you will mess up and turn her off.

When you set up the date, suggest a good date idea and give her 2 options for days. If she agrees to one, set it for that day and lead by telling her when and where to meet. If she is vague and doesn't seem too interested, leave it for now. Act unaffected and like it's no big deal to you. Ping her 2-3 days after and try again. If she's still not showing interest, let her go.

When you do set up a date, text her a couple of hours before to remind her, and tell her that you'll be 15 minutes late. This will give her an opportunity to tell you that she can't make it. She'll only do it if she was already thinking about it; you're just bringing it up to the surface. You're saving yourself from wasting time and showing up to nothing.

If she does flake on you and lets you know in advance that she won't show up, don't be reactive. Act as if it's nothing. Don't ask when she's available next. Let her chase you. If she doesn't, then you don't have much chance with her. Think abundance and let her go.

Your main focus should always be on becoming a more attractive guy, not on getting that one girl.

We hope that you found this eBook helpful on how to turn a number into a date. Remember that your mindset is more important than the specific wording of the text. There is no magic line if you're not an attractive guy, to begin with. Having said that, when you are an attractive guy, having good phone game will help you and increase the chances that she'll come on a date with you.

Thanks for reading this book. I really hope you enjoyed it, and if you haven't yet, could you kindly leave this book a review on Amazon?

I really appreciate your review. Thank you.

How to Talk to Women

A Simple Guide on How to Talk to Women If You're Shy and Never Run Out of Things to Say

Sabrina Shuman

Introduction

Men, we need to talk. No, I don't mean that literally. Let's analyze the situation for a moment: Why does it seem like all our sisters and female friends get teased by grown men? And why do they accept the abuse without ever fighting back?

It all comes down to one thing: communication. There are many ways to communicate with women besides just words; we disregard this fact and instead focus on what they say or how they look. It's time for us to grow up and become more mature in our relationships!

Here is a list of things you can do that will help you to understand women better:

1. Ask questions. It doesn't matter if the subject is about work, food, or your life; it's important to have a basic understanding of the other person's life. Example: "How was your day?" "What did you do today?" "Where are you going next weekend?" You can also use this opportunity to make small talk. Example: "Did you like that movie?" (Start off with a compliment.) "...Yeah, I saw it too." (Keep on talking) ...how was the movie?... ohhh... interesting. So, what did you think about it? Ohhh interesting...I was wondering if you can tell me what the movie was about?... ohhh, interesting. That was

cool ...ohhh, interesting...Thank you for the compliment. How are you today? Ohhhh interesting...So, how are your kids doing?... oh, WOW, that's amazing.... you have a family? Oh, I didn't know that! Thank you! Have a good night. (Talk more about yourself)

If one day she answers with "I'm fine" or "Don't worry about it." You will start to wonder if she really is fine.

2. Avoid telling her how hot or beautiful she is. I know guys are insecure, but hear me out first. It's not a great idea to tell them they are beautiful. This is because they have been told that their whole lives, and sometimes it has been said in a negative way (think about when someone calls you ugly). Instead, compliment her on her personality traits and let her know that you're genuinely curious about her. Example: "You are very confident" or "you look like you're having a great time!"

3. Avoid cliché' lines like "where have you been all my life?" or "you are the most beautiful woman I've ever seen." These may work for some guys, but if you want to stand out from the competition, avoid using cliches. Instead, use your own creative and unique style.

4. Compliment her attributes she wouldn't expect you to notice (like her sense of humor or how well-spoken she is). When you are listening to her, focus on the things you like about her, and don't be afraid to compliment her! Let

her know that she has something special and that you like it! This makes a much stronger impression than telling someone they look pretty. Remember: You want to be honest with women.

5. Be a gentleman. I'm not saying that all women want a man who opens the door for them. But, be respectful of other people and how they feel. If you have a problem with a woman, don't just come out and tell her. Instead, ask her for advice on how to handle the situation. It helps if you get her genuine thoughts on the matter and what she may have experienced in a similar situation. This also makes it more personal instead of just throwing out random insults like "why don't you stop being so lazy and do the dishes!"

6. Be yourself around women. Don't go out of your way to impress women with how much money you make or how manly or masculine you are (this will only make them feel uncomfortable). Instead, be yourself! Be friendly! If you are that confident, they can figure that out on their own.

7. Focus on the conversation. The wickedest thing you can do is to try and keep the topic about yourself. Don't feel that you have to impress them with your stories or say really obscure things just to make them interested in you. If the woman doesn't seem genuinely interested in what

you are saying, stop talking altogether and ask questions about her instead. This is about getting to know each other better and not just being self-absorbed!

8. Pay attention to her presence. This should be obvious, but don't look around the room when she is trying to talk to you or start playing with your phone as soon as she enters the room. Just because you are confident that you are good-looking and smart doesn't mean that women have to act the same way. If she seems more interested in talking to other people, relish on your confidence and look for her at a later date.

9. Actively listen to what she is saying (or put yourself in her shoes). This goes along with number four above, and I said it first, so don't be rude about it. If she says, "I love this restaurant," agree with her. Don't say, "yeah, I like it too!" Why? Because then she will assume that you're just saying that because you really like the place or that you're trying to show off to impress her.

These are just a preview of what you can learn from this book. We will also talk about attraction and flirting with women in-depth later on. But there are many great tips in this book that can really help you take your game to the next level. Let's begin.

Chapter 1:
How to Talk to Women

D o you find yourself a bunch of nerves while talking to women? Does approaching the fairer sex become a big issue when you're doing it for the first time? Are phenomena like stuttering and mumbling common while you are trying to 'score'?

Well, the good news here is, you are not the first one, and definitely not the only one. Here I will guide you through some commonly witnessed and fairly successful tips to follow if you want to talk to the Eve-descendants without getting your nerves in a twist:

1. Eye contact is usually the first step to breaking the ice. Make sure your eye game isn't too bold or too feeble. Put in as much effort as you would to just about let her know that you have a mild interest in her. Too strong eye contact shows you in a bad light, and so do too mild ones. Remember, it's glancing and not staring. Know the difference between the two.

2. If there's anything common between missile launching and dealing with women, it's the right timing. Knowing when to strike up a conversation is a good card up your sleeve. Women are usually organized and all scheduled

up. Anything or anyone that tends to disrupt their timetables is seen as undesirable and often ignored. Choose intervals of time when her attention isn't distracted toward others and more important stuff. Also, timing is as much about 'how long' as it's about 'when.' Be on guard as to when you are exceeding your time limit. There's no such objective limit, but you ought to know when you've run out of your quota.

3. If you are new to her, it's advisable to take the first step with a neutral compliment. Compliments can be tricky. If delivered in the wrong manner, they can backfire almost instantly. For example- ''you always look good in that top'' is a disastrous compliment to give to a woman you're meeting for the first time. It implies you've been stalking her. Start with a very casual yet sweet one like, ''you're smiling a lot today. What are you so happy about?''. A good compliment is one that leads to a conversation. Don't hang around awkwardly after showering truckloads of compliments on her. Compliments are launch-pads; they can only spark up the fire. The rest needs efforts.

Another thing to be kept in mind while attempting compliments for a woman is that body and figures are strict no-no areas to start with. Talk about her smile, her hair, and her eyes and mandatorily avoid talking about her body, however hot she might be. Most women, despite their open-mindedness, do not approve of their bodily statistics being talked about in initial conversations. Wait for her to open herself to you and until she does, play it safe and smooth.

1. To successfully strike a conversation, you also need to pay attention to your body language. Women have been known to be reluctant to talk to guys with short attention spans manifested by flickering eyes and twitchy feet. On the other hand, a patient posture and a cool attitude work wonders in establishing a decent first impression.

2. What most guys do not pay attention to is their personal hygiene. If you're the advocate of the "Guys are supposed to be like that" ideology, then chances are the woman you are pursuing has already made up her mind about you. Women like their seekers neat and hygienic. It necessarily doesn't imply they don't dig the bearded and the shaggy, but there need be a line drawn between tolerable and distasteful. Clean nails, trimmed face, and neat clothes go a long way in conveying your hygiene. It also doesn't mean that you need to go all metro-sexual and be the brand ambassadors of creams and pedicures. All you've got to take care of is some basic sprucing up. Sweat pants and loose Tees cannot work wonders a decent tucked-in shirt and a pair of seemingly dry-washed jeans can.

3. Most guys don't know how to kick-start a conversation. If you're a goner with compliments, then you could try ice-breaking through asking favors. Asking a menial favor that doesn't require much investment on the woman's part is a solid first step. ''Could you fetch me that pen?'', ''Hey, what date is it?'', ''Can you press the lift button for me?''. If you're shy to be asking favors, then you can try making a statement! This is the safest weapon at your disposal. ''I love the coffee here'', ''the weather today just sucks'' etc.

Make a simple statement, expressing what you believe is valuable or worth getting concerned over, and roll out the ball in their court. If the woman is interested, she'll pick up the statement and continue it with her own thoughts and opinions on it. If she doesn't, then you were simply making a statement. No loss.

4. Always strike a balance between casualness and graveness. Too much of either is a turn-off in most cases. Generally, women like their Johns and Toms to be a perfect blend of happy-go-lucky and a serious attitude. If you're too casual about things, you're presumed fickle. Same way, if you can't talk about patriotism without citing historical references of freedom struggle, then you are probably someone a woman would avoid after the first conversation. Show her you are versatile by

changing approach-gears according to the situation and its demand.

5. Know when a woman is not interested in talking. Such knowledge prevents you from making an embarrassment out of yourself. Most of the time, one can always tell whether a conversation is receiving the woman's approval or not.

Overcome Shyness

The first step to talking to people is getting over your shyness. Many people suffer from shyness, which can range from occasional episodes to debilitating shyness that often gets in the way and keeps people from doing meaningful things in their lives. It is usually considered a form of social anxiety, which can be overcome with practice.

Beginning to overcome social anxiety starts with determining the reason why you are anxious in the first place. More likely than not, the underlying cause is that you feel self-conscious or that you will be automatically judged. Some people become so anxious about how they will be perceived by others that they find it hard to even get out of the house. The bad news is that if you think you're automatically going to be judged, then, to an extent, you're right: once you physically enter someone's sight, you will be under scrutiny.

The good news is everyone else is being judged too. You yourself are guilty of judging people by their appearance. It's our nature. Nobody is immune, which puts us all on the same playing field. Also, every single person has things about them that make them feel self-conscious. It may be how they look, how they speak, or how they walk, but there is always something. Lots of times, what we think are glaring imperfections about ourselves are barely noticeable by the general public and are definitely no reason to hide. If there is something obvious about you that makes you uncomfortable, just own it. If your big nose makes you uncomfortable, pretend it doesn't. Unless you plan to have plastic surgery, you might as well get used to living with that nose. Life will go on either way.

Don't be afraid to talk to other people. They are likely just like you, and they may have the same social anxiety. Think about the last time you were at a networking event. The essence of those events, especially in business, is meeting new people and creating new connections that can further your career. Everyone at these meetings tends to find themselves in the same boat: they all talk themselves into going and promise themselves they can leave after talking to five people. Honestly, everybody has the same social hang-ups and anxieties to deal with. Nobody really wants to go, but they do so anyway to better themselves and their business.

At these events, didn't you feel relieved when someone came up and started talking to you? That person had to take the brave step to overcome social anxiety, walk over, and start a conversation. They didn't know you or have any idea what they could be walking into, but they did it anyway. Next time you head to a marketing event, make someone else feel comfortable by making the first move. Initiate the conversation and just see where it takes you.

Sometimes the only way to overcome shyness is to pretend you are confident. While you may feel jittery and nervous inside, it may be necessary to put on a brave face as you try and conquer your fears. Don't worry, it will get easier. Remember that social grace is not just something people are born with; it is an acquired skill. It takes practice to feel comfortable speaking, so just as you would schedule a tennis lesson, plan in time to work on your social skills.

If you feel uncomfortable, mentally remove yourself from the equation. Think of yourself as an actor. Your role is to play a confident, knowledgeable business person who is marketing themselves to a new group of clients. You are not a shy, inexperienced person straight out of college; you are a seasoned professional with hundreds of clients under your belt. Now, act that way.

Just take a step and put yourself out there. Socializing and talking to new people will feel scary at first, but as you learn and improve your skills, each new situation will become easier. Talk yourself into following through with new situations, regardless of how overwhelmed you feel. Practice positive self-talk to motivate yourself and give yourself the confidence you need to follow through. Those who have developed better social skills often say that overthinking is the root of their social anxiety. Very analytical people tend to look at a situation from all possible angles, including all of the bad ones. Giving focus to potential problems arising in or because of a conversation lowers your confidence, making you want to avoid the conversation altogether.

For example, you are due for a promotion at work. At your yearly assessment, you plan to deliberate the pay increase and new responsibilities with your boss. You know this meeting will happen at the end of the week, giving you more than enough time to prepare. A confident, socially adept person will practice what they plan to say, including all of the reasons why they deserve the raise. Others will overanalyze, considering all of the things their employer may say to try and deny the raise. While it is a good idea to be prepared for a possible downturn in conversation, focusing on the negatives of the conversation before they happen can be a killer! By the end, you will have successfully sabotaged your own good intentions and talked yourself out of your raise before your boss even has a say.

Instead, leave only a little time for thinking about the possible downsides of your argument. Don't dwell on the negatives; consider them briefly and find a way to turn them into positives. That way, if it does come up in conversation, you will have a good way to respond. Instead, put all of your efforts into planning for the positive and boosting your self-confidence.

Chapter 2:

What Women Want in a Man

I 've always heard that women are really complicated to figure out. I have to disagree.

I think you need to start with the fact that every woman is different, and you need to embrace that, but I've learned in my experiences with them what they want when talking to men.

The Top Ten Qualities Women Say They Look for in a Man

1. Confidence
2. Sense of humor
3. Reliability and honesty
4. Not a pushover
5. Intelligence
6. Resourcefulness
7. Passion
8. Ability to communicate
9. A protector
10. Physicality/attractiveness and sex appeal

So, let's break these down.

Confidence

It just keeps coming back to this, doesn't it?

Women love confidence. It's sexy and pulls them in. Remember, there is a difference between confidence and cockiness. Confidence is often unspoken, more of a vibe than the actual words. It's in the way you stand and the way you speak. And women can't get enough of it.

Sense of Humor

Having a sense of humor isn't just about telling a joke but also about not taking yourself too seriously. If you tease her, she's probably going to tease you back. In fact, you should hope she does because that's a sign she's flirting back and interested. So, don't get easily offended.

It's one thing to let a joke slide off you, but if you actually got insulted, make sure you don't get angry and just let it go. Although, it might be time to walk away. Remember your self-worth. You never should allow someone to insult you.

Many times, the woman won't even realize that she said something that offended you. Just like men, women sometimes gest without meaning any harm. When you point it out to them, they will apologize and back off. This shows that you are often willing to stand up for yourself without having to fly off the rails, and she will respect you more. But if the woman tries to brush off your concerns or acts indignant for being called out on it, then you need to walk away.

Reliability and Honesty

Women don't like liars. It doesn't matter if you lied to them about cheating, what you do for a living, or that you are wearing clean socks. They want to know that you are telling them the truth.

They also want to feel that you are reliable. From the first time they meet you through dating and sometimes into marriage, they want to know that you will be there for them and do what they ask and that you promise.

A classic example of this is the "Honey Do" list. When you are in a relationship, there will be things that she asks you to do, from errands to household chores, and a lot of times, couples call it the "Honeydew" or "Honey Do" list.

Some boyfriends and husbands don't take this list seriously, but it's a way to show that you are dependable. Make sure you are constantly checking things off and getting them done. Believe me, she notices.

Not a Pushover

You don't have to be over-demanding by any means, but you need to stand up for yourself. Don't let people (or her) walk all over you. While you want to do things for her, you aren't at her beck and call. You have a life and goals of your own.

Intelligence

Once, a woman was telling me about a guy she dated who was extremely handsome but not too smart. She told me a story about how once they were watching television and "bookends" were mentioned in a joke. Her boyfriend just looked at her, not understanding. She proceeded for ten minutes to try to explain to him what bookends were. He still had no idea. She finally got up, went to a shelf, and grabbed a pair to show to him. He laughed and said he didn't know they had names.

To make it worse, one day, he was looking at the spices in her cabinet and started asking what things were while he mispronounced them. The woman told me that at that point, she knew the relationship was doomed. She would even tell the guy, "It's a good thing you're handsome." And he still didn't understand she was insulting him.

Women want you to have a brain in your head. You don't need to be a rocket scientist, but you need to know how the world works and how you fit in. And always learn how to pronounce the names of spices.

Resourcefulness

Women love a guy who can figure stuff out without sweating. It can be something as small as changing out a broken light bulb with a potato (look it up!) or finding a way to get tickets to a sold-out   concert.

Women love that you can figure it out, especially when you have the ability to figure it out for them. It makes them feel special.

Passion

Women want a man who is passionate about things, and they know when you are serious.

It needs to be passionate about important things. First of all, they want you to be passionate about them, but they want to see it in the way you talk about work, family, and even hobbies.

Be forewarned, though, if your hobby is volunteering, she's going to be more impressed than the passion you express when, say, you gush over your baseball hat collection.

Ability to Communicate

Women want a man who knows what he wants and can put it into concise words. It doesn't matter if you are ordering a sandwich or talking to her about a relationship.

Women are constantly complaining that men don't open up to them. This is a bit misleading to men. They think that women want them to open up the floodgates and let emotions and feelings out.

Now, you don't need to bottle up everything, but they aren't looking for an hour-long session of telling her your innermost thoughts and feelings. She really just wants you to be honest and   tell   her   things.

As men, all too often, we are taught to bottle things up and carry on. Many men are told to hide their emotions and bottle them up. They think that they shouldn't show off their emotions. But how can that help when you are trying to relate to another person?

Be honest. If something is bothering you, tell her. If there is something in the relationship you aren't getting (even sexually), tell her. How is she going to know if you don't tell her?

A Protector

Women want to feel safe. You don't even have to do anything but let them know you are there for them.

It's going to be different with different women, too. I need to mention here that I am pretty tall. Once upon a time, I dated a woman named Lauren, who was a former model and about 5'10". I also dated another woman named Kate, who was about 5'5". They each wanted to feel protected, but in different ways.

Kate loved that I was so much bigger; she could get lost in my arms when I wrapped them around her. She would tell me how secure it made her feel and that when she was with me, she felt safe.

Lauren, on the other hand, didn't need to feel physically protected in the same way because she was so much taller. Heck, she was taller than a lot of guys out there. But she told me she felt safe as well for different reasons. She said she felt as though I had her back. That she could take care of herself, but just in case she didn't, she had me as a backup. She called us partners in crime.

Protection isn't always about being big and being able to physically sweep her away from danger. Sometimes it's more emotional and psychological.

Physicality/Attractiveness and Sex Appeal

Of course, she needs to be attracted to you physically, but did you know it can be a lot more than how you look that attracts her to you? It's actually a combination of all the above things.

True, some people just aren't going to be attractive to others, especially if you don't take care of yourself externally, but it's so much more.

By being her protector and making her feel safe and cared for, you are triggering primal urges in her brain. Going all the way back to the days of the cavemen, women are biologically wired to find the best mate. While part of that is physical attractiveness, their brains are wired to look for the man who can provide her with the best offspring, protect her against danger and other men, is trustworthy, and always comes home to take care of her.

So, when you show her that you offer these other things, it builds her attraction to you on a primal level.

Here are some things that are useful to do:

Find Out What Interests Her

So, how do you show her how you fit into her categories?

Well, it's not just as simple as rattling down the list and telling her which things on her checklist you qualify for. She wants to know exactly how, and she wants to discover it.

So, you need to do some work. You need to organically see how you fit in and then show her where you match and have connections. She needs to find out that you are the right guy, but you definitely need to help it along.

Ask Her Questions

During a conversation, women love it when you ask them questions. The problem is that a lot of guys don't know how to ask questions.

Make sure you ask real questions that will reveal something interesting about her and follow up.

Turning around from a Dead End

If you ask her something and the answer is a dead end, sometimes you can turn it naturally.

You may have just gotten back from a great vacation and have a good story to tell, but you ask her if she likes to travel, and she says, "not really," you probably don't want to tell that story. So, what do you do? Turn it.

"So, you must do a lot locally. Any cool places I should know about?"

See, it's turning a negative into a positive and pushing the conversation forward.

Don't Go On...And On... And On.... And On....

If you are telling a story, don't go on for everything. Don't dominate the conversation. Conversations are about give-and-take and back-and-forth. If you are doing all the talking, she's going to get turned off.

Don't Be Cruel

Women like a little teasing, but everyone has their limits. Always be aware as you are finding that limit and don't fall into cruel or mean jokes.

Chapter 3:

Approaching and Flirting with Women

B efore you can engage in a conversation, you must be able to start one.

Luckily for you, there are billions of women on the planet. So, it's not difficult to find one to start a conversation with.

And yet, so many men have trouble with this.

Why? Well, it's a combination of fear and insecurity.

They're afraid that women will reject them – and, even if they somehow make it through the first part of the conversation, they're afraid that they'll run out of things to say.

And so, they rarely initiate conversations. As a result, they don't meet nearly as many women as they should.

So let's tackle that fear of approaching...

You're in line at the supermarket. You look over to the next register line, and a beautiful woman catches your eye.

You admire her hair and her style, and you smile for a moment – she's exactly your type.

"Credit or debit?" the cashier repeats to snap you back to reality, and you hand her your card. You sign the receipt and grab your bags – but when you look back at the woman, she's gone.

"Damn!" you think to yourself. You missed your shot. But as you walk out the door, you see the same woman walking right in front of you.

You clam up for a second, wondering if you should make your move or let her go...

The excuses start flooding your brain... "She probably has a boyfriend..."; "She's a little too tall for me anyway..."; "She looks like she's in a rush..."; "I'd have to catch up to her to say 'hi' and that feels weird..."

What do you do next?

There are three possible scenarios:

1. You listen to your excuses, do nothing, and let her go.

2. You approach her, and it goes well.

3. You approach her, and it doesn't work out the way you wanted.

I was in this exact situation the other day. At first, I succumbed to my excuses – and I felt terrible about it.

But when she stopped on the street corner for a minute, I swallowed my pride and went for it.

The result? She gave me a big smile, and a minute or two later, I walked away with her phone number and plans for drinks later that week.

I felt the fear but did it anyway.

So – what was going through my head then – and what can you do to propel yourself forward when you're afraid to approach her?

How can you start seizing the opportunities instead of letting them slip through your fingers?

It comes down to the following 4 actions...

Focus on Overcoming Your Fear

If you're afraid to approach her, it actually works in your favor.

You see, boldly confronting your fear can feel far more rewarding than simply starting a conversation with a random woman.

One of the greatest discoveries a man makes, one of his great surprises, is to find he can do what he was afraid he couldn't do. – Henry Ford

When you focus on confronting and overcoming the fear, you'll not only approach more women, but you'll also grow as a man.

You'll realize, "I had these excuses. I had this story I was telling myself. But I approached her anyway. I did what I was afraid I couldn't do– and it will feel awesome."

Shift Your Perspective

Often the reason you're afraid to approach her is that you feel like it's too risky. She could reject you and damage your ego. Or maybe she'll respond well, but then you'll run out of things to talk about.

In that moment, these fears are perfectly reasonable. It's easier and more comfortable for you to do nothing than to take action. The risk of rejection and embarrassment doesn't feel worth it.

When you're afraid to approach her, your risk spectrum looks like this:

Risk of approaching her: You'll have an awkward interaction, get rejected, and feel terrible – a big risk.

Risk of doing nothing: No risk – you'll save your ego, stay in your comfort zone, and move on like nothing happened.

But you need to shift your perspective so that it's actually more risky not to approach her.

You need to adjust your understanding of the risks, so it looks like this:

Risk of approaching her: Potential awkward interaction with a woman you'll probably never see again. So, 1-2 minutes of discomfort – a small risk.

Risk of doing nothing: You miss out on a potentially amazing connection and incredible sex with a woman you're attracted to – a big risk.

Risk of building the habit of not approaching: You signal to your subconscious that it's "okay" to not approach women you're interested in. In doing so, you miss out on other great women in the future – another big risk.

With this perspective, it's riskier for you to do nothing than to approach her.

Use this reversal of risk to propel you forward and get the women you want. Make a conscious effort to view approaching women from this perspective.

Stop Waiting for the Right Moment

Don't waste time waiting for the right moment. You won't find it – you'll always have an excuse in your head as to why it's the wrong moment.

Instead of waiting, make a habit of walking towards the woman you want to talk to. Don't comb your brain for the perfect thing to say, and don't pause.

Just start walking towards her.

She could be talking to her friend, on the phone, eating lunch at an outdoor patio – it doesn't matter. If you don't talk to her now, you probably won't get another chance – and if you wait too long, you'll build up the fear in your head and psyche yourself out.

As I always say, if you point out a woman and tell me to approach her now, I can do it – no problem. But if you point a woman out and tell me to approach her in 5 minutes? Well, that's a whole different ballgame. It's going to be A LOT tougher because I'll be building it up in my head for those five minutes, as opposed to if I just took immediate action.

So, take the first step. The action will help you conquer the fear.

Listen to your excuses and, in the end, let them go.

Tap Into Your Manhood

Why do you want to approach her? At some level, she gives you the feels. You find her sexy and intriguing.

But often, you leave your attraction on the backburner and instead focus on the fear of approaching.

All of these thoughts start going through your head. "Does she like me?" "Should I try to kiss her?" "What should I talk about?" "What if she thinks I'm boring?"

Instead, you need to keep your attraction and appreciation for her beauty at the forefront of your mind. This will help you cultivate a nervous excitement instead of nervous fear—an excitement to meet and learn more about her.

How do you do that?

Ask yourself: What do you like about her?

Do her eyes draw you in and captivate you? Is her smile contagious? Is her rhythm sexy? Does she make you laugh? Bring these thoughts to the forefront of your mind.

As you appreciate her inner and outer beauty, you'll be more in tune with your natural male instincts.

For me, it always brings a smile to my face and leads me to make strong eye contact. It allows me to be more free-flowing and in the moment as well.

When you approach her with this excitement, often she will mirror you. Even if she isn't into you at first, she'll begin to find you intriguing and feel the same type of excitement.

So, tap into your manhood and focus on what you find attractive about her – this will make it easier to approach, and the woman will usually respond better.

Listen, man, the fear of approaching a new woman will always be there. You can never completely eliminate it. But that's okay – you don't need to.

A little fear is what makes the process fun and rewarding.

So, keep these four actions in mind to help you conquer fear when you feel like it's overwhelming you.

To recap, here are the four actions for overcoming your fear of approaching her:

1. Focus on overcoming your fears

2. Shift your perspective

3. Stop waiting for the right moment

4. Tap into your manhood

Ways to Start a Conversation With Any Woman

You now have four concrete actions to conquer your fear of approaching women. But once you approach them, what do you say? How do you start the conversation?

Well, what you say to start the conversation depends on a few things, like:

- The environment. The way you start a conversation during the day may be slightly different from how you start the conversation at a nightclub.

- The woman. If she's in a rush, you'll have to move the conversation quickly. Whereas, if she's standing and watching a street performer, you know she has some time, and there are plenty of things to talk about.

- Your goals. Maybe you're not super interested in the woman and just want to build some social momentum. Or, maybe your intuition literally forced you to talk to this woman because she caught your eye so strongly.

Whatever the situation, this will help you start the conversation well and move things forward with the woman.

(Keep in mind – when you're in a naturally social environment, like perhaps a social sport, house party, or a get-together with new friends, you can be pretty casual with the way you start a conversation. That's because it's expected to be social in these types of situations.)

Chapter 4:

Body Language, Mind Games, and More Techniques for Conversation with Women

D id you know people meeting you for the first time form an impression about you in the initial four seconds? Hard truth? You bet! If you want to go from being a weekend Netflix binge-watcher to a guy who is never short of dates, you got to be a dude who creates a stellar first impression. If there's one secret sauce or magic potion when it comes to wooing a woman, it is creating a powerful initial impression.

Deep research into the science of seduction reveals that attraction isn't confined to a single domain. It is a combination of neurology (NLP), psychology, sexual studies, and evolutionary science, which is why I am revealing the ten most super awesome tips when it comes to sweeping a woman off her feet in the first meeting.

Grab Your Place under the Spotlight

Guess what? Even though we have evolved from our primitive existence, our subconscious mind is still deeply hard-wired in its patterns when it comes to relationships and social gestures. There's a reason we still mark our territory physically and subconsciously, and entering our space leads us to act in a more territorial manner.

Well, okay, no one's asking you to come into the limelight by acting weird or hyper-energetic. One way to demonstrate confidence when meeting a woman you desire for the first time is to take your own space. Don't be the nerd who fades into the background while others hog center stage.

You don't want to stand out for the wrong reason, but that doesn't mean you don't get noticed (which is equally bad if you ask me).

Own your zone and take up your space immediately. Expert tip for owning your space – seize up space within 3 feet as your own private space. Think of yourself as owning that private bubble and ensuring any woman who passes through it has a great time. Focus on completely owning the space around you, and you'll have the gathering's hottest gals noticing you.

Some body language and seduction experts suggest taking as much space as you can. If you are seated in the lobby, lean behind and spread out your legs. This is a subconscious, territorial instinct that women notice. Well, in the woman's mind, if you are occupying a lot of "territory," you are the room's alpha male—the one who is in command, as well as fun, confident and laid-back.

Create an Emotional Rapport

The journey from meeting a woman to taking her to bed becomes surprisingly easy when you build a powerful emotional rapport with her. Psychologically, mirroring is one of the most effective ways to forge a strong mental connection with the woman you desire. Start mirroring the way she stands, speaks, holds her glass, and gesticulates.

Keep it discreet, and don't make it look like you are stalking her. Subconsciously, mirroring sends the other person a message that you are pretty much like them and makes it easier for them to connect with you on a mental plane. Gradually mimic her posture or use the same words/phrases as she does. Once you practice this strategy, it will come effortlessly.

For example, if the woman holds her glass on her left side, try and hold your glass of drink on the left side too. If they are making a particular gesture with their hands, try and make that gesture too for conveying that you identify with what they are trying to communicate and acknowledging the same.

Mirroring works wonderfully well because it is seen as something beyond the realm of our conscious awareness. When you repeat someone's actions and words, you secretly send signals of familiarity to them through the subconscious.

Seduction boy language experts suggest that you should mirror or mimic a specific gesture three seconds after it is first noticed.

This lets you imitate a person without them freaking out or becoming suspicious about your behavior. Although, on the surface, you are simply mirroring the lady's body language, the end goal is to match her feelings, views, thoughts, and yes – maybe even the breathing pattern. Even minor actions like posture, expressions, blinking, verbal acknowledgments, and scratching should be matched. If this technique is implemented correctly, the woman will fall for you like a pack of cards!

Another quick way to build an emotional rapport is to reveal a vulnerability in the correct manner. According to research, some women take to weaker men. However, weakness is also a relative trait. Remember to never make the blunder of revealing low value and terrible weaknesses. This may really go against you. For example, you may want to narrate a sob story related to your ex, but this will only make you look like a cry baby who cannot move on.

If you are using this psychological trick, ensure you pick your weaknesses with care and don't opt for weaknesses that make you look cheap or unflattering. Instead of concentrating on your past, build emotional rapport via future projections. How about an exciting thing you've fantasizing about all your life? Talk about an exciting travel experience that's on the top of your bucket list. Just reveal some fun thing without overdoing it. You are doing nothing but controlling the woman's mind without making her realize.

Women possess a way more powerful and vivid imagination than men, which makes them see the exciting things in their mind's eye. Also, you've shared a personal dream or goal with her, which makes you instantly adorable to her. Practice this technique regularly, and keep watching for the body language of couples who are already in the rapport-building stage. You'll witness amazing results in little time.

Open Up

You don't want the woman of your dreams to think you're a closed, secretive, and guarded person. Of course, you don't want to come across as a sparrow on steroids, but keeping an open and approachable demeanor works to create a glowing first impression.

I'll let you in on all secret body language strategies to appear warm, open, and approachable. To begin with, keep your palms facing upwards (open and exposed). Remember how you reveal all your cards by flashing your palms upwards in a game? Well, you aren't exactly revealing all your cards here. However, you are demonstrating a more "open to you baby" kind of demeanor.

Another big cross on the list of things to avoid is crossing your legs or arms while standing or sitting. Even if you don't realize, it has "closed" written on it in bold. You are psychologically blocking yourself from your wonder woman.

Another vehement no-no, if you're holding a drink, don't hold it right in front of you. Hold the glass down, sideways.

Master these little known techniques that most men don't have a clue about to enjoy an edge over them when it comes to garnering attention from the opposite sex.

Hide your feelings by all means but, but keep the hands open. Also, displaying a lightly off-the-limits or playing hard to get body language doesn't hurt. You need to keep a fine balance between not acting too distant (will make it appear you aren't interested) and not acting too eager (which makes you come across as desperate).

According to research conducted by Timothy Wilson and Erin Whitchurch of the University of Virginia, acting slightly indifferent towards women can lead them to contemplate your distant behavior, and eventually, develop a liking for you.

Be Attentive

Women don't take it kindly if they are relegated to secondary status. If you fancy them, they should be the center of your world. Don't move around or act fidgety around a woman you desire. Preoccupation and distraction are a huge turn-off. You're not giving off a very flattering vibe to the object of your desire if you make perpetually fidgeting and nervous gestures. A man who controls his body language will be taken more seriously than one who is awkward with his gestures and movements. Keep your feet slightly apart while sitting, which will prevent you from constantly shifting your weight from one side to another.

Shifty, fidgety, and distracting gestures are a huge sign of nervousness that takes away from an essentially calm, confident, and relaxed demeanor, which you want to portray.

Don't make too many confusing gestures that send the woman you desire perplexing non-verbal signals. Twitching your body excessively or making too many animated hand gestures is an absolute no-no. It gives off the feeling that you aren't very comfortable with your body and leaves a damp first impression. When you appear uncomfortable with your own body, how do you expect women to be comfortable near you?

Of course, you don't have to be all over the woman and shower her with unwanted attention. That's a huge no-no too. Acting a little indifferent to things happening around you is alright; just don't act too fidgety and distracted. Cool indifference is mighty appealing; nervousness is not.

A majority of men falter here. They believe it's cool to act all busy and distracted to impress a woman. So, what does Mr. X do? Whip out a smartphone from his pocket and pretend to be occupied with important matters. What does it reveal to the lady? You're simply not interested enough to give her undivided attention. Well, don't blame her for getting the impression that you want to be somewhere else.

Instead of appearing distracted, keep all objects of distraction away and appear interested in your immediate surroundings. Keep your body language alert, focused, and aware of your environment. Put your head up, and relish the moment, which makes you appear more approachable. Plus, you pick up all the silent, non-verbal invitations/signals women stealthily send you.

If you really want to score with a woman, avoid showing too much emotion or reaction to things happening around you in the first meeting. Display a more unaffected demeanor. Let others play the guessing game about how you think and feel. This makes the challenge of getting to know you up, close and personal even more compelling.

Stay at the top of your dating/seduction game by showing you are always in control and relaxed. Everyone loves people who own the situation.

Flaunt the Sexiest Voice You Can

Ever wondered why women are attracted like moths to a fireball to men with deep, husky, and low-pitched voices? Women are essentially auditory creatures who are instantly attracted to a calm, strong, and controlled voice/tone.

Talk too fast, and you'll come across as nervous. Speak slowly, and you'll run the risk of appearing dumb. Keep your tone steady, unwavering, and well-paced. Make a conscious effort to make yourself audience and clear by speaking slower than you usually do while talking to a woman. It will award you greater control of what you're saying (plus you'll time to think about what you're going to say next).

Avoid stressing about mistakes and stammering during the conversation. Even if you do make a mistake while speaking, cover it up by saying something humorous quickly to salvage the situation. Think and speak according to the situation.

Something like, "Ah! Damn, this is exactly what happens when you're in the company of sweepingly attractive women. You totally forget what you want to say." This will not just be flattering to the lady but also make you come across as high on wit and humor. Self-deprecating humor is a sign of huge confidence.

Sometimes while talking, pause for a moment and appear serious. This creates an aura of power, influence, and confidence.

Chapter 5:

Dating and Sex with Women

I t's what we are all looking for, right? You may be the type of man who needs it almost every day and will be happy to have sex with any woman, or you might be a bit more selective for physical or emotional reasons. It doesn't matter. Eventually, we all want to have sex. I'm guessing that's a big reason you picked up this book.

Know Your Sex Ed

It's hard to believe, but it seems like there's an increasing number of men who either didn't pay attention in sex ed classes, had cruddy ones, or were exempt from them altogether. They don't seem to know a lick about female anatomy, sex, or safe sex. Some of them barely know about their own anatomy.

I remember talking to this one guy on Twitter who genuinely thought that women could hold their periods in and choose when they happen. Seriously. He thought that feminine products were unnecessary because they could just "wait until they got to the bathroom if they wanted to." I am perfectly comfortable in my masculinity and gender identity, but that is the closest I've ever come to being ashamed of being a man.

Please, brush up on your sex ed before actually hitting the sack with someone. Why is that important? Because if you don't understand how it works, there is no way that you'll actually be good at it. Even if you know roughly what will make you feel good, if you don't understand or properly remember sex ed, you won't be able to figure out what will make her feel good. Trust me, it's a lot better when you can both enjoy it.

Women will also be more attracted to you if you know your stuff in this area. It might not come up often in conversation, but if it does, looking informed is the much better option. Otherwise, you don't look like just a moron; you look like a misogynistic pig.

Safety First

Okay, guys, you've had this drilled into your head since you noticed your first woman. Be safe. You don't want to catch something or, even more, have little versions of you running around out there. In all seriousness, part of being a real man is acting responsibly and protecting yourself and your partners. Be a man.

Condom

Always wear a condom unless you are in a committed relationship. Even then, make sure that you have talked about birth control and your thoughts on what to do if the unexpected happens.

Get tested regularly. Even if you practice safe sex, get yourself tested regularly for sexually transmitted diseases.

Don't Believe the Myths

There are some myths about ways in which you can keep a woman from getting pregnant without protection. One of the most prominent and well-known ways is called "pulling out," in which the man pulls out right before the big moment. The problem is that there's no guarantee that this will prevent pregnancy. In fact, there's no proof that any of a number of myths will work. Since you're a grown adult, I suggest cutting through all of the hooplas and just going with the tried and true: condoms, birth control, sponges, and other kinds of contraceptives.

No Stealthing

"Stealthing" is when a man will put on a condom at the beginning of sex, often at the woman's request, and then remove it sometime during without telling her. Often, the woman won't find out until she finds out that she has an STD or is pregnant.

Now, most men won't do this. It's a cowardly and jerk thing to do. Still, there are a few men out there who will try and make women distrust all men even more. Just because it feels better to you without the condom does not mean it's the right thing to do. Think about the big picture, and respect the woman you're with enough to wear a condom if that's what she wants.

Putting It in Isn't the Only Way You Can Catch Something

This isn't the most fun topic, but the cold hard truth is you can get diseases from oral sex, both giving and receiving. Probably the most common of this type is herpes. While it isn't sexy, take into consideration using condoms or dental dams during oral sex.

This is one of those reasons to start talking to women about sexual history before sleeping with them. You have to make an effort to protect yourself with knowledge.

Virginity

It's also possible that you picked up this book and you are a virgin. You have never had sex before and don't know what to do, expect, or how to proceed. What do you do to get the opportunity to have sex? Is something wrong because you haven't yet?

First of all… nothing is wrong with you. There are people who have stayed virgins for years and those who lost it when they were teenagers. Everyone is different.

Is It a Choice or Circumstance?

Some people make a choice to wait to have sex until it's with someone they care about or love or maybe even until marriage.

It's a personal choice, but honestly, a lot of people make it in their teens or early 20s and then end up changing their minds.

If you think you are a virgin by circumstance, that you can't find a woman who will have sex with you, that's garbage. There will always be a woman out there who will have sex with you. Always. The question is, do you want to have sex with her? I'm guessing there have been numerous opportunities for you to have sex, but you probably didn't realize they were out there. It's not circumstantial; it's a choice you made.

Should You Tell the Woman?

This is a tough one, but my initial answer would be no, with a caveat.

I don't believe that you should volunteer the information. It shouldn't come out in conversation. "Well, I was born in Boston. I like football, oh, and I'm a 26-year-old virgin."

Yeah, not a good idea.

However, if it comes up naturally and you feel a connection with her, it's ok to tell her. But don't dwell on it. Don't tell her you feel strange about it or that you are missing something. Just say the right opportunity hasn't come up yet and leave it at that.

I would highly suggest that you tell her after the fact if you didn't already. You don't want her to think that you are inexperienced. She will actually be happier to know that she is your first and will actually want to have sex with you more to teach you what she knows and see what you can learn together.

What if I'm Bad at It?

Sex is not anything like you see in the movies. You always see it go perfectly; no one pulls on each other's hair, no one puts things where they shouldn't go, everyone looks great afterward.

Sex can be messy, full of mistakes and problems even with the most experienced participants — especially the first time together. So, don't worry.

Can She Tell I've Never Had Sex?

Well, the sure way she'll figure it out is if you tell her.

For the most part, no, she's not going to know. In fact, most guys who have little experience tend to brag more about it. And women know this.

As for the actual act, odds are she's going to be a little nervous because it's your first time together. She wants to have fun but most likely has her own insecurities and fears. So as long as you don't do something fundamentally wrong, like trying to put it in her ear, she's not going to be worried it's your first time.

She may think you are inexperienced (which you are), but as I said above, you should tell her afterward.

But What if You Know... It's Over Really Quickly?

It sucks. And it happens to every guy.

Be honest with her. Explain it was your first time. As long as you don't get weird or cry or something, she's going to understand. And if she doesn't, it's ok. Her real personality is showing, and you see it.

If you notice it's becoming a problem, then you might need to start working on your technique or mental place in order to make it last longer. Try different positions and ways of having sex that doesn't push you toward the end so quickly. You can always think of baseball scores.

Honestly, when you get more experienced and are with someone you have a connection with, you will last just the right amount of time.

Initiating Sex

Sex usually just happens. It isn't planned, at least by the couple. It's usually just when the build-up is right; the time has come.

If you are already kissing and moving toward it, then just let it progress. However, at some point, she may push back. Be very aware of what she is saying to you.

When She Initiates It

I will admit, sometimes we men can be a little oblivious when women are the ones trying to initiate sex. Women can be much more subtle with their advances. When you combine that with not wanting to make any assumptions, women's advances can go right over our heads.

Shortly out of college, I started seeing an older woman named Miriam. We didn't sleep together right away, so I figured that Miriam wanted to take things slow. On the fourth date, she invited me to her place since her sons were with their dad for the week. After dinner, we snuggled up on the couch to watch a movie on Netflix. We kissed a bit but nothing too serious. Suddenly, Miriam draped her leg over mine, causing her short, short dress to ride up. Then, she started running her hand over my chest. The nail in the coffin—what really should have driven her point home—was when she gave me a kiss on the neck. And what did I do?

Nothing. Just like a moron, I smiled at her, kissed her forehead, and returned to watching the movie with her all over me. Fortunately, Miriam, being an older woman, knew not to play these games long and finally just kissed me full on the lips. Things progressed naturally from there.

Afterward, Miriam admitted that she had been trying to "seduce" me (her words), and I admitted that I had no clue at all. After we shared a good laugh at my expense, Miriam shared one of many valuable lessons that she taught me in our relationship: most women will be subtle about sex. They'll be sensual, she explained, not overtly sexual.

Chapter 6:

Being Her Sweetheart, Boyfriend, and Even Husband

A ct Respectfully When You Are With Her.

First, I'll change the title. Be respectful at all times. This goes back to the kindness bit. Don't talk shit about her to your friends. If you both keep your fights and arguments between just the two of you, your friends and family won't have a skewed opinion of the person you love most. Because we always seem to forget to tell them when we SO apologized.

It says to open doors, pull out chairs, give her your jacket when she's cold, all that stuff. I'll add to that. If she opens the door for you, just walk through it. If she wants to pay, just say thank you.

It says to pick your clothes more carefully and have proper hygiene. Hell to the yes!

Avoid any offensive actions in public, like swearing or belching. Okay, I'm obviously not the one to tell you not to swear. Or belch, for that matter. But do edit yourself in public on both accounts. And do I really need to add farting? I mean, I get that it happens, but try to make it the silent but deadly type and blame it on the dog. Although she'll know after a while. And if you have to rip a loud one in public, at least make it funny. Once, when I was subbing, I dropped a silent one as I walked past the popular kid. I was like, "Duuude!" I don't know if he was still popular the next day. I was just the sub. Not my problem.

Carry her books and backpack for her between classes or after school. Okay, I'll call bullshit on this one. If you're in high school or college, you have your own shit to carry. If you're an adult not in college, it's moot. But the whole damsel in distress bullshit is sexist. Like we can't take care of ourselves. Yeah, a lot of women play up that stereotype.

Compliment Her And Be Genuine About It.

Don't take the bait when she's fishing. Instead, call her out. Say something like, "I know you're fishing, and I don't want to take the bait. Wouldn't you rather my compliments be sincere?" Then make sure you sincerely compliment her. They don't all have to be about her looks, either. I gave you a bunch of compliments to choose from earlier, but here are a few more. Be sure to compliment her on the things she's most self-conscious about. If it is about looks, be specific. Like, "I love your crooked nose. Seriously. It adds character." "I think the gap in your teeth is adorable! I really do." "You really don't need bigger boobs. They're perfect for me. Besides, you don't want the back problems those other women have" (she really doesn't). But let's give a few examples not about looks. Because you're thinking of her now, aren't you? You're thinking of the tiny little details about her that you know/ think/ fear she hates- her freckles, her weight, her hair, her height- you're thinking of it because you do find it adorable, amirite? Tell her that. Moving right along.

- I love your laugh. It's adorable. It makes me smile.

- I love the way your eyes light up when you talk about...

- I love the feeling I have when I see you like everything's going to be okay.

- I love the teamwork we have when we do this...

- I love coming home to you.

- I love waking up to you.

- I love your smell.

- I love you even more than your dog.

<Okay, don't out and out lie. That's not even possible.>

- You're really good at...

- You're really smart at...

Let Her Know She is on Your Mind

You don't need to text her all day, and you don't even need to respond immediately. If she's an actual adult, she'll get that you're busy. She is too. But text her at least once a day with more than, "Sup?" Ask a specific question about her day, or send an inside joke, or just say, "Hey, just thinking about you. Hope you have a good day." Women find that cute, and if it's not all day long, you're a fully functional adult with a job and a life. But if it's at least a little bit, they'll still be an important part of that life.

Surprise Her with Romantic Gestures

Yes. Do this. An article I read suggested a playlist of songs that remind you of her. Yes. Do that. If you have an "our song," it needs to be first. Do not include Stupid Woman or You're a Bitch or any rap song about stupid ass hoes. You're welcome.

The article also suggested slipping love notes into her locker. Okay, we're talking about the long haul here, people. The M-word. Or at the very least, the F word. No, not the Fuck word. We can get that anywhere—the Future word. Yeah, high schoolers know who they want to marry, but they have no idea how to do their taxes. Or that they'll need to.

The love notes are a good idea, but if you're in high school, focus on your studies, kid. Just throw a few in her car's console someday. Put some in your hoodie pocket. The hoodie you know she's going to borrow and never return.

Ask to borrow her car someday. Return in fully washed, with a full tank of gas and a dozen roses on the seat. She'll rave about that for months.

Do these as preventive measures instead of fixes. It's a lot easier that way.

The list suggested getting her something she can wear every day to remind her how much you care. Okay, no. Was this written by a man? Men don't know how to shop for women's clothes. They barely know how to shop for their own.

I'll give a few suggestions of real ones. The love notes and playlists are good. My car wash idea is good. Here're a few more.

- Notice what's in her fridge. Bring her groceries based on her tastes occasionally.

- Send her a book about her celebrity crush.

- Randomly put money in her PayPal.

- Buy her surprise gifts from Amazon. Everyone likes surprise presents! Stuff she'd like, maybe body spray and lotion gift baskets, movies she hasn't gotten around to buying, pictures similar to the ones hanging in her house already.

- Plan a picnic someplace unusual- the mountains, a rooftop, the bed of a truck.

Have Fun & Make Her Laugh

Yeah, everybody likes to laugh. Include plenty of banter in your relationship. Don't get all butthurt if you walk into one and she picks it up. Be disappointed in her if you accidentally lay 'em down and she doesn't pick 'em up. If she walks into one, ya gotta take it. Them's the rules.

But make sure you don't tickle her if she doesn't like it. Make sure you're not making fun of her for something that actually hurts. When she tells you to back off, do.

The two cardinal rules: treat her like she's human and back off when she says to; that's not just about sex. They're for all the time. If she says she doesn't want to talk about it, try believing her instead of forcing her to talk when she's still upset, and her words won't come out right. Just back off.

Chapter 7:

Picking Up Women at a Party

A woman can tell when a man is checking her out, and when she catches him checking her out, he often looks away. What he should and must do is smile at her and immediately approach her. A woman's radar is always in active mode, and she can usually tell when you're interested. If you hesitate, you project weakness and uncertainty. If she senses weakness and uncertainty from you, you've already lost.

Over 50 percent of Earth's inhabitants are female, and just about all of them (within reason) are available to you. We no longer live in the Victorian Age, where women were ruled solely by their reproductive systems, and marriage was the most significant event in their lives. When it comes to courting and relationships, modern society is more open-minded than ever. Although there are some notable exceptions, there is no longer a class system, and pre-arranged marriages are rare. We can unexpectedly find love and happiness at any age, at any time, and in any place. You have more choices than at any time in modern history, and you have the liberty to choose the woman that you want and desire. Most importantly, you have all the time you need to meet and fall in love with the woman of your dreams.

When Should You Approach?

The correct answer is always (unless she's a grieving widow at her late husband's funeral). If you spot a woman you want, you must boldly approach her immediately. The problem for many men is that they approach women with an attachment to a hoped-for outcome, and they start to make assumptions on how they should conduct themselves during the initial contact with her. Here's what I mean: "That woman is pretty, and when I make my move, I hope that she'll like me. I have to say the right things and then she'll give me her number. I have to take her on an extravagant and expensive date and impress her enough so that she'll have sex with me and want to be in a relationship." Many men live by these incorrect assumptions because they're suffering from a scarcity mindset or the negative influences of social conditioning.

Because many men fall victim to social conditioning or have a self-defeating, scarcity mindset, they often have crippling attachments to getting laid and roping her into a committed relationship before she's ready. They'll often come off to a woman as inauthentic, needy, or trying-too-hard and cause her to lose any interest she may have initially had in him. Small mistakes during the pick-up stage and early dating stage can have big consequences. These are the men that consistently lose the game right from the first pitch. They're out.

Here's what you should be thinking: "That woman is really pretty, and I'm going to go and talk to her and see if I like her. If I like her, I'm going to make a firm date with her right on the spot, or I'm going to get her phone number right on the spot." Why? Because I have an abundance mindset, and that's what always happens when I approach women. Women always give me their phone number, and they always agree to a date.

Logically, you know that's not what will always happen. The magical panty-dropping, over-rehearsed, scripted, pick-up lines that you may have read about simply won't work with healthy, accomplished Alpha Females. Try some lame-ass, cheesy pick-up line with a quality female, and you're going to get rejected. But if you have an abundance mindset and always speak your truth authentically from your heart, your approach will be much easier, and rejection won't be so damn painful. You must have the mindset of, "I always get what I want, and if I get rejected, it's her loss."

Another mistake that many men make is they disqualify themselves before they've even attempted their approach. Here are some examples: "I'm probably not her type...She's with her friends...I'm too short...I'm too tall...I don't make enough money...She probably has a boyfriend...She's busy...She's stuck-up...She won't be interested in me...etc."

Really? You know all these things about her before you've even spoken to her?

Here's what's happening: Such men internally rationalize their unwillingness to approach a woman because they become terrified of getting rejected again. Humans naturally seek to avoid pain (such as the pain of rejection) and engage in activities that are more likely to bring immediate pleasure or a sense of safety. It can be difficult for us to do something that involves risk. Approaching a woman you find desirable creates the possibility of a long-term, loving, and mutually beneficial relationship with the woman of your dreams. But with your approach comes the risk of rejection, and there's no way around it. The risk of rejection is always present when you approach a woman, and the hard truth is that you will get rejected sometimes. I'm going to talk about how to overcome approach anxiety and your fear of rejection as we proceed.

Read Her Tells

Wikipedia defines a poker tell as: "...a change in a player's behavior or demeanor that's claimed by some to give clues to that player's assessment of their hand. A player gains an advantage if they observe and understand the meaning of another player's tell, particularly if the tell is unconscious and reliable."

A woman will exhibit varying degrees of positive body language when she's interested in a man. Positive (or negative) body language is her tells, and, like Wikipedia's definition, her tells are usually unconscious and reliable. When you're able to read her tells properly, you'll have the advantage. When she's interested, her face, torso, and feet will all be pointing at you. When she's interested, she will often lean in towards you and will often put herself in your personal space, almost touching you. These and other tells are a huge part of understanding and correctly reading her degree of interest in you. The more you practice reading feminine tells, the better you'll become at reading feminine tells. Should you determine that she's not interested in you by correctly reading her negative tells, wish her well and politely move on. If she's not interested, there's nothing you can say to change her mind because attraction cannot be forced. Cut your losses and move on.

Of equal importance, the body language you display will have a big impact on causing her interest in you to grow or diminish. Excessive positive body language from you shows too much interest too early and will sabotage your game. Remember, small mistakes at this stage can have huge consequences. To avoid appearing too eager when meeting her for the first time, turn your body, so you're standing obliquely to her vs. head-on. As the interaction continues, let her see that she's merited your interest by presenting more positive body language by gradually turning more fully towards her. With that in mind, here are some of the most common feminine tells to watch for:

Mirroring Tells: As you're conversing with her, her body language may begin to mirror yours. For example, she may stand the way you stand, she may place her arms in the same position as yours, she may take a sip of her beverage when you take a sip of yours, etc. When she unconsciously begins to mirror your physicality, she's feeling a connection and is comfortable with you.

Open Posture Tells: When she's interested, her body language will be open, she'll face you completely, and she'll unconsciously position her head, torso, and feet to point in your direction. She may not display an open posture right away, but as you continue engaging her properly, you'll notice her body language opening up to you. Tilting her head to the left or right and exposing her neck is another open posture tell. However, if her head, torso, and feet continue pointing away from you, her interest in you is low or nonexistent, and she's looking for an escape route.

Leaning Tell: If she's becoming interested in you and she's enjoying the interaction, she'll begin to lean towards you and that's true if you're sitting next to her or across from her or if the two of you are standing and conversing. When she starts to lean in towards you, you've aroused her natural, feminine curiosity, and you now have her full attention.

You spot her leaning tell by giving her the space that she needs to lean in. That means you don't lean in at all. You're not aloof or arrogant, and you're giving her all of your attention, but you're not projecting eagerness by leaning in. If you're standing, just maintain a relaxed posture. If you're sitting, lean back, relax, and take up space. Always give her the space that she needs to grow her interest in you naturally and at her leisure. If she leans back, no big deal, just let her lean back and allow the interaction to progress naturally. When she's ready, she'll again lean in towards you. Be cool, and don't crowd her.

Touching Tells: Playfully hitting you, accidentally brushing up against you, or briefly placing her hand on you are all tells that she likes you. For you, properly touching her is also a good way to increase her interest in you. But tread lightly. Touch her too much, too early, and she may begin to feel uncomfortable. A good rule of thumb is if she touches you playfully and briefly, you return the same touch playfully and briefly. When she touches you, it means she's green-lighting you to reciprocate. In fact, she may unconsciously want you to touch her in return. Start with a light, brief touch on her upper arm or her shoulder or the small of her back. But again, tread lightly. You must always give her the freedom she needs to become ever more comfortable with your touch, and she may start to crave your touch. While touching of any sort is a sign of interest, the more intimate the touch, the higher degree of interest she has in you. A woman touching your chest or thigh is showing a higher degree of interest than if she's just touching your arm or shoulder.

But remember, this is your first encounter, and small mistakes can have big consequences. If you're unsure, don't touch her at all.

Chapter 8:

How to Talk to Women: Secrets of the Alpha Male

C onquer Your Fears

To be an alpha male, you have to learn to live your life to the fullest.

Alpha males have mastered conquering their fears of the unknown. They have learned to embrace discomfort just to pursue something they are passionate about. They know there will be challenges in the pursuit of their goals, but they are still willing to do it.

Write down the things about life that you're afraid of. Consider every area where fear is holding you back from living your life to the fullest.

Probably you've become overweight, and you're afraid that people will ridicule you when you go to the gym. Or maybe you are stuck in a toxic relationship, but you're afraid that if you get out of it, you'll never find another woman to love again.

Whatever it is, write it down. When you're done, ask yourself these questions:

- What could be the worst thing that could happen?

- What could be the best thing that might happen?
- If I fail, how long does will it take until I'm back on my feet?

You'd be surprised that when you think about what you were afraid of, the worst outcomes may not be as bad as you thought they would.

Get out of that comfort zone and live!

Don't Let Anyone Tell You What Path to Take

Alpha males have a clear vision and purpose. They know what they want to do with their lives. That is how they inspire others. They know what they want, and they don't let others dictate to them where they should go to pursue their goals.

Chart your own path, then take action. Fulfill your destiny.

Aim for Constant Progress

For alpha males, their true competition is themselves. They will never get caught wallowing in self-pity because other people are more successful than him. They don't compare themselves with other people.

Success may not yet have come to them just yet, but they know that small successes will eventually bring them to their ultimate goal.

So, don't worry if your life is not as good as your friends. Success in life doesn't happen in an instant. It's a process, and you have to go through the process to appreciate your success more.

Don't Argue Just Because

Alpha males believe in action and learning rather than starting a disagreement. They wouldn't waste their time arguing about their beliefs, religion, philosophy, and politics on the internet or with their circle of friends. Instead, they are committed to taking action on what they know will help improve themselves.

This doesn't mean that you should shy away from intelligent conversations and debates. The key is to agree to disagree.

Do Good Because it is the Right Thing to Do

Alpha males are kind and have the deepest desire to do good. But they are not doing this because they want to become popular, but simply because they are good people.

They help people without expecting anything in return.

They have genuine compassion and empathy for others.

They believe that the only thing that matters is the impact you had on other people.

When you wake up in the morning every day, ask yourself this question, "What good can I do today?"

Always Speak Your Truth

When alpha males believe in something, they won't hesitate to defend that belief.

The alpha male speaks his mind but still with respect for others. They will not back down from anything they believe in. While he may respect the opinions of other people, he will not be controlled by these opinions.

Speak your mind even if other people might shut you down. Be brave enough to stake a stand.

Develop Self-Reliance

The alpha male is his own man. He cultivates self-reliance. He knows he has the power to make his own choices because they know it is the best option.

But to be self-reliant doesn't mean you shouldn't ask for help from friends or neighbors. There will be instances when you need to admit that you need help.

Build a Strong Body

You don't have to have six-pack abs or 20" biceps to be considered an alpha male. However, you should be both physically and emotionally fit so you can build a strong body. You have a responsibility to yourself and to others to take care of your well-being.

You can't live life to the fullest if your body is not strong and healthy.

You Should Know How to Defend Yourself

To be able to defend yourself. You have to be physically fit, so this ties back to the last habit. Every man should learn to fight at some point. Little self-defense techniques would suffice, though.

Take Care of Yourself

Self-care is important, especially if you're an alpha male. Your well-being should be a top priority.

Start with one act of self-care a day. You may try meditation. Or one day you can try to do something you enjoy doing, like a hobby. Go to a sauna or get a massage.

So, don't neglect your health.

Live by Your Values

You should live by your own code. Define your values and live by them. Live with integrity.

Most people develop depression and anxiety because they are living a life that is not aligned with their values.

Don't say your family is important, yet you spend more time working. To have a happy family life, you should spend time with them.

Do you want to be happy? Then all that you do, all that you say, and all that you think should be aligned with one another.

Establish what's important to you. If it's family, then go for it. If it's financial success, then pursue it. If it is to go on an adventure on your own, then go. You don't become less of an alpha male if you pursue these things.

Be True to Your Word

Your word is your honor, so you have to keep it. If you say you'll do something, then do it. If you say you won't do it, then don't. That's a straightforward principle.

Keeping your word gains the trust of the people who follow you. Your reputation would also be good. But most importantly, you learn to trust yourself.

Your words are important, so use them wisely.

Failing to live up to your word will become easier for you to lose conviction. Whatever you say won't have an impact anymore because no one will believe you if you keep on failing at your promise.

You're human; you get exhausted, so don't spread yourself thin. Give promises that you know you can keep. If you are unsure, then do not commit. It's better to say "no" early than to break your promise later on because you didn't have the luxury of time.

In this modern world, it's hard to find a man who remains true to their word no matter the circumstances.

Don't be one of those men.

Master the Art of Charm, Attraction, and Seduction

You should be able to attract certain types of people who can help you to achieve your goals. Likewise, you should also find a woman with whom you can build a family with if settling down is one of your main goals.

Improving your confidence would help boost your charisma.

Make Your Life Harder, Taste Sweet Victory Later

You have to understand that alpha males do not hope to make an easy life; their main goal is to grow, not to live in luxury and comfort.

They know that the challenges and adversity they'll encounter will make them stronger. These will help build their character and teach them to be resilient. Make the uncomfortable your new comfort.

You Have to be Willing to Die for Something You Believe in

Alpha males are willing to die for anything and anyone they love. They will die fighting for their family, their honor, to defend their values, etc.

Becoming an alpha male is no easy feat. It's a journey; it doesn't happen overnight.

You might have to encounter discomfort and hardships or suffer pain, but it will be worth it in the end.

Chapter 9:

How to Talk to Women Online and by Email

T alking to women online can be overwhelming. As a guy, there's an inherent fear that you'll come across as creepy and will scare them away before you get to engage in any meaningful conversation. This chapter will teach you the best ways to talk to women online without putting your foot in your mouth or coming across as creepy. Here are some guidelines you can follow:

Stick To One Topic

Most online dating sites have a "message" section which is where you can talk to women without having them think you're an ax murderer. Before jumping into the "message" section, make sure that you've decided on a general conversation topic, such as hobbies or interests or favorite movies.

Use Specific Subject Lines (Like Online Dating) And/Or Ones that are Complimentary ("Wanna Cyber?")

Another thing that will help you get a woman's attention is using an appropriate subject line whenever you send your message. Never use the title of the book, like: "Hi there." That doesn't really mean anything. Ask her if she wants to cyber or if she has any questions. You can also give a compliment; just don't make it generic. For example, if your message is: "You have beautiful eyes," she'll probably think you're one of those guys who are being nice because they expect something in return. If you want to compliment her eyes, then tell her why you find them beautiful. You can say: "Your eyes remind me of the ocean." That's telling her exactly why you like what she has, and it makes for a more interesting conversation than just saying that her eyes are beautiful.

Respect Her Privacy

If a woman demands that you do not contact her, respect that request and try someone else. Women aren't desperate to meet men, and if they don't want you to contact them, then respect that.

Keep It Brief And Simple

This is another rule you should follow when talking to women online: keep it brief and simple. If she asks about something she's interested in, tell her a little about that subject before going on to something else. You can also ask her whether she enjoys the subject matter or ask for her opinion. There are plenty of ways to transition from one topic to another without making your message look like a disorganized mess of random thoughts.

Keep It Casual

Another thing you want to do when interacting with women online is to make sure that you're responding casually. If she wants to know about your job or your family, it doesn't mean that she's trying to dig for information about your financial status or trying to find out if you're actually married. She's just interested in what you have to say and wants a general idea of what your life is like.

Be Supportive

One thing that most women appreciate is a man who is supportive of their ideas and interests even if he may not necessarily like those exact same things. For example, if she tells you that she's a big fan of indie rock, don't say, "Ewww, I hate indie rock," because it'll make her think that you hate her too. Instead, just say that you've never really listened to that genre of music before, but you're willing to listen to some of her favorites and see if you like it. Whatever it is that she loves, be the kind of guy who accepts her for who she is and not who he thinks she should be.

Don't Use Too Much Slang

If you're using too much slang or internet lingo, then it'll make your message look silly and unprofessional. Stick with the correct grammar because a lot of women appreciate a man who's intelligent enough to type correctly.

Be Unique

This is another extremely important thing: make sure that your message isn't generic or boring. If she asks you a question and you respond with a generic answer, then what's the point of even talking to her because your responses aren't going to be interesting enough to keep her around. Think of this as a chance for you to be creative. There's no reason for you not to come up with something that's unique and interesting, whether it's a compliment about something she mentioned in her profile or an inside joke that only the two of you know about. It does not really matter whether you make your message more interesting, just as long as it is.

Don't Tell Her Everything About Yourself

If she asks you something specific, tell her exactly what she wants to know without going into too much detail. Just make your answer short and sweet, and don't tell her too much. Any more than that will just appear as if you're trying to monopolize the conversation, which will also be unappealing to her.

Don't Overdo It

If you're on a first message, then don't open the floodgates right away. If she asks you about your travels or about something you did last weekend, save those for the next message or even the next day if she's interested in learning more about your past experiences.

Keep It Brief, But Do It Well

You should not want to make her think that you're interested in her message because you're messaging her all the time. She'll probably respond to your messages before you've even read them, but if she doesn't, then don't worry about it. Just make sure that every time you message her, whether she replies or not, that your message is short and sweet. It provides us a sense of urgency to respond and makes us curious enough to do so.

Be Enjoyable

If your message isn't enjoyable for her, then she'll just delete it without reading it because surely she has more important things to do with her time than send messages back and forth with someone who's not interesting enough.

Make Her Feel Special

If you make her feel like she's the only woman in the world, then she'll be more likely to keep on talking to you. This doesn't mean that you should lie about how many other women you're talking to or what you've talked to in the past. Just be honest about your situation and tell her that she's a special woman to you and that she deserves your best efforts in making her feel important.

Show Off Your Personality

Always think about how much effort it took for her to create a profile on the site, and take the time to go through all of the information on there before messaging her. Chances are that you're going to get a response from her, and if she doesn't, then she might not stay around long enough for you to take an interest in her. The more effort that you put into your message, the better chance that she'll respond with one of her own.

Be Genuine

Don't try too hard just to impress her, or else it will seem as if you're trying to converse with her, which will turn off many women on the site. Just be as genuine in your attempt at getting her attention as possible, make yourself appear as though you don't care whether or not she messages you back or reads your message at all. It will become easier for her to respond with something.

Be In Charge

If you're the one who is doing the pursuing, then you'll be in the power position, and she'll feel more feminine for being the pursued than she would if she had to do all of the chasing. Just remember that you should never ask her out on a date or try to set anything up at this point because it will make you look as though you're desperate and that you have nothing to do other than messaging her.

Don't Try To Persuade Her To Meet Up With You

Women don't want to be persuaded to do things that they don't want to do, so if you do this, then she might be able to tell that you're trying too hard and that it will scare her off. She'll feel as though she doesn't have any say in the matter and that she's being coerced into doing something against her will, which will make her feel less feminine than she would if she had taken a little more time out of her day to message you first. It will also make it seem as though you're so desperate for a date with her that you'll do whatever it takes, which is not exactly attractive.

Take Things Slowly

This one is very important. Whenever you would want to establish a relationship with her, or even if you don't simply want to get to know her more, there are several ways you can show interest. Making an excuse to go out for dinner, texting her only in the morning when she's awake, or sending her a text at random times throughout the day are all ways to get your foot in the door without making it seem like you're too desperate or needy. If she has time during her days off, then take advantage of that and initiate contact with her.

Respond As Soon As Possible

Don't wait a week before you respond to the receipt of one of her messages because it will make you seem completely disinterested and give you less of a chance to actually get to know her. You want to respond as soon as possible, whether that's in the next 5 minutes or the next 30. The sooner you do so, even if your message is just "ok" or "cool," the better off you'll be.

Chapter 10:

The Right First Impression

"**I**t is better to be first in a little thing than to be last in a great work." -Confucius

Making a great first impression is one of the most important things you can do with your dating life. When you mess up in other areas (e.g., your pictures or profile), a girl will still open you and give you a chance to make it right. However, if she doesn't like the way you come across in person, then most girls won't even give it a chance and simply swipe left and never look back.

This is one of the main reasons so few guys have success, and why even if you're in the 99th percentile as far as your looks go, you can still struggle with online dating...your personality came across poorly.

Because of this, it's the NUMBER ONE thing I stress with my clients: to make a good first impression. And to get that good first impression, they have to nail three areas:

1.   How You Look

2.   First 1-3 minutes talking (The Attraction Phase)

3.   Body Language

1.   How You Look

If you're a decent-looking guy, this is perhaps the least important of the three. However, if you're a particularly "ugly" guy (meaning you're in the bottom 20% or so but seem like an awesome person), then this will be the biggest thing you focus on.

That being said, you still want to make sure you're attractive enough, but not so much that it becomes a burden. You also don't want to approach like some kind of supermodel, getting all self-conscious about your looks and not giving off any personality.

In fact, what I call "The Rule of Threes" is important here: you should always be looking for at least one other girl in the picture (other than yourself), even if she doesn't stand out too much. It may seem counterintuitive (why would you bother?), but the point is to NOT stand out TOO MUCH.

For example, let's say you're a guy in a picture with your friends. However, you're the prettiest one in the group. Yes, you may get some extra attention and swipes from women who like your look, but the fact that there are other people in that picture will make it seem normal that some girls swipe left as they think it's only about looks and not about personality. On the other hand, if you're by yourself in a picture, then it becomes much more about looks. So, you want to be somewhere in between—to show that you have good looks but not so good looks that it seems like your card is based solely on your appearance.

As for clothing, you should dress like you're at a normal photoshoot. You don't want to look like you're on an episode of Project Runway. Instead, it should feel more like a typical date: casual, but not too casual. Women are generally looking for guys who dress well and don't look like they just got out of bed.

2.   First 1-3 Minutes Talking (The Attraction Phase)

Here, you want to make sure she's attracted to you. You do this through your body language and the way you talk.

You should be standing in a position where you are facing her when talking so that she is able to read your facial expressions and see if you're smiling or laughing during the conversation. You don't want to be sitting down, as it makes it much harder for her to get a sense of whether she likes you or not (unless, of course, it's at a café or bar).

When she sees that you're smiling at her, she'll feel good and will want to smile back. If she doesn't, she might just swipe left without even starting the conversation. Of course, you want to be pleasant even if it seems like nothing is happening. But that can take time and effort in a conversation, so start out on a strong note (i.e., humor) so that women can feel good about talking to you right off the bat.

If you're the one who starts the conversation, then step in front of her when doing so. This takes away any awkwardness and makes it seem like you know what you're doing. Then you can walk a few steps with her and say hello.

The BIGGEST mistake men make here is not making the first move and being too nervous to start talking to a girl. They stand around for five minutes before they work up the courage to approach—which by that point, is way too late.   When talking, don't be dull and boring as most guys are on their first date. Make sure there is some sort of fun or humor in your game (e.g., if you're going to the zoo, say you like giraffes and then say, "If I had a choice in the matter, I'd want to be a giraffe!").

You also need to make sure your jokes are good enough so that she will laugh at them. If she doesn't laugh at your comment, then it probably wasn't "funny enough."

3.   Body Language

One of the biggest mistakes guys make is their body language. This means everything from the way you walk to the way you sit. And even though I'm not a body language expert, I can tell you that there is an easy way to improve where you are, what you're doing, and how you look.

First off, always stand in a position where she can see your face. This is why men talk over women during conversations and why they have their arms folded—so they can look down at the girl's face. It may seem like this might be a good thing, but in order for her to feel good about talking to you, she has to feel like she is looking into your eyes when talking. Plus, by doing this, you're better able to flirt with her since your eyes are a powerful pickup tool.

Two things you can also do here:

i.   Stand in the way so that she has to go around to get past you if she wants to go into the venue or whatever space you are in. This is a simple move and will help heighten the intensity of her emotions when talking to you.

ii.   Make sure that your arms aren't crossed over your chest (unless it's cold out). Instead—like I mentioned above—you want them hanging freely at your sides. Doing this will make you look open and approachable and will make it easier for her to talk to you as well.

Another big mistake guys make is walking around with their hands in their pockets. This makes you look like you're not interested in the girl or don't care about what's happening. Even if that is the case, it doesn't help your cause if she can clearly tell that you don't think talking to her is important.

Instead, keep your hands always visible by either putting them behind your back or holding something (e.g., a bottle of beer).

Doing this will give you a more open look and will make you seem more appealing to her.

Lastly, when you're talking to a girl, make sure that your body is turned towards her (and not the other way around) so that she feels like she is the focus of your attention. In fact, I recommend turning 90 degrees to your right then walking towards her while talking. That way, when you are done with one topic, you can simply turn left at an angle and talk about another topic in that same pose. This kind of back-and-forth works well for creating attraction and is a very easy move for anyone to practice.

Chapter 11:

Be a Charming Conversationalist

Y ou see the beautiful woman. You swallow your pride, walk up to her, and make a great first impression. She responds well.

Yes, that sexy woman is intrigued by you. But to build a connection, you need more than just a solid approach. If you don't carry the same energy and intent into the rest of the conversation, she'll lose interest.

It's not as complicated as it may seem though. She's rooting for you. She wants to have a fun interaction with a cool guy—and you're that cool guy. Now, you just have to deliver.

Here's how to do it:

The Question/Statement Balance

Have you heard of 'interview mode'? It's when a guy starts rattling off question after question to a woman like he's interviewing her.

He runs out of things to say, and he gets lost in small talk. So he lets loose with all the old classics...

"What's your name?" "Where are you from?" "What do you do?" "What school did you go to?" etc. etc.

She's had this conversation millions of times. It's boring. And remember: this isn't college anymore. You don't have the same baseline of trust with women that you did back in school. If you rattle off boring, interview mode questions, women will wonder, "who is this guy, and why does he want to know my life story?!"

But, if you want to build a connection, it helps to know these things about a woman, right? So you need a way to learn more about her and infuse excitement into your small talk.

Behold the power of statements. You can turn almost any question into a statement and tease the woman in the process.

Here are some boring small talk questions you can replace with statements:

Question: "Where are you from?"

Statement: "You look like a Jersey woman. "

Question: "What do you do for work?"

Statement: "Okay. Let me guess—you're an accountant. I can totally see you crunching numbers all day."

Question: "What's your name?"

Statement: "You look like a Susanna. Just have that old school, southern belle vibe."

With statements, you make a guess about the woman, and she gets curious about your guess. She wants to know why you think she's a Jersey woman or an accountant. And this presents the perfect opportunity for you to tease her. You learn more about each other, have fun, and avoid entering the dreaded interview mode.

Think of some more common questions you'd ask a woman and write them down. Then, write some possible fun statements that you can make instead. Get into the habit of thinking, "How can I turn this question into a statement?"

Statements work because they help you get past small talk—and this is crucial because small talk only serves one purpose: it's a jumping-off point into getting to know each other. The longer you remain in small talk, the more social pressure builds, and the more awkward it gets.

Here's an example of a typical small talk conversation. You've probably had a similar conversation at some point.

"Where are you from?" you ask.

"I grew up in New York and moved here after college. You?" she says.

"I'm from Rhode Island."

"Oh, cool," she says. "What do you do?"

"I'm a lawyer," you reply. "I work at the courthouse downtown. How about you?"

"I work at the entrepreneurship center at the state university," she tells you.

"Nice," you respond. After a short, uncomfortable pause, you ask, "So, how do you like working in the entrepreneurship center?"

"It's great. I love working with students. What about you? How do you like being a lawyer?" she asks.

"It's okay. Gets boring at times, but it pays the bills," you say. She laughs politely, and then there's another awkward pause—this one, longer than the first.

"Well, I should go find my friends," she says. "It was fun meeting you."

"Nice to meet you too," you say.

Could you feel the social pressure ramping up? You never got past small talk, and the conversation died out. It got more and more awkward until one of you had to leave.

You both missed opportunities to have a real conversation and genuinely get to know each other. The conversation remained superficial. Even if you both like each other at the outset, this kind of conversation will destroy any chance for a good connection.

To get past the small talk, you need to make statements and balance those statements with the right questions. You must listen carefully and relate to her, so you both can reveal more meaningful information and you can actually get to know her. Here's an example of how the above conversation could have gone differently:

"You look like you're from Jersey," you grin.

"Why do you think I'm from Jersey!?" she laughs.

"You just give off that Jersey vibe. I'm starting to feel more guido just talking to you."

"Hahaha, no!" she says. "You're ridiculous! I'm from New York. What about you?"

"I'm from Rhode Island, the Ocean State. Mermaids everywhere. I love New York, though. I've had some crazy adventures there. What made you leave there for Boston?"

"I went to college in Rhode Island!" she says. "But I fell in love with New England, and then I got a job offer at the university entrepreneurship center after I graduated. Couldn't pass it up."

"Haha, me too, what school did you go to?! And I'm really passionate about entrepreneurship. I feel like that's the only way to make your mark on the world!" you reply.

"I feel the same way! And I love working with the students and helping them with their businesses…"

Do you see how this conversation is different? Instead of rattling off interview mode questions on autopilot, you make statements and then relate to her answers. The conversation turns from boring and predictable to fun and exciting.

Here are some other examples of questions that help you relate to her and build a connection (notice how these aren't just yes or no questions. These questions require a more thought out response):

- "What do you like about that?"

- "Why did you decide to do XYZ?"

- "What's your most epic story from XYZ?"

- "If you could do anything else, what would it be?"

- "How was it growing up there?"

When you listen, relate, make statements, and ask questions like these, you'll break conversations out of autopilot and build great connections. Women will feel like you know them well, even if you've only talked for a few minutes.

Be Unfiltered (And Never Run Out of Things to Say Again)

There will be times when you're at a loss for words, even if you listen and relate to her.

Whether you're at a loss for words, or you just want to make the conversation more fun and move it to the next level, being unfiltered is key.

If you can master this concept, you'll never run out of things to say again. You'll avoid awkward silences, make the first move without hesitating, and have tons of fun interactions.

To further emphasize this point, here's what a couple of my past coaching clients had to say about being unfiltered:

"Dave's central theme of being unfiltered can literally create changes in the responses women give you overnight. When I say this, I mean, once you have figured out how to be unfiltered, you will notice immediately that women and others respond to you in a more positive way."

"You're not going to believe this, but I finally got a number and a date using your methods. I just sort of said fuck it, I'm going to say what I want to say, be it awkward or not, and it worked!"

So, how do you be unfiltered?

Well, have you ever wanted to say something but stopped yourself short because your brain told you it was risky...maybe even inappropriate?

Say that thing.

Instead of saying the safe thing, you say what's really on your mind.

You make random statements and observations about the environment. You make innuendos on a whim. You tell jokes because YOU think they're funny—not because you want a woman's approval. In fact, you don't even care about the woman's reaction. If she thinks it's funny, that's cool. But if not, you're still self-amused. And if you want to tell a woman she is sexy, then you tell her straight up.

Basically, you say whatever is on your mind, even if it doesn't make sense. The result will be ridiculous and unpredictable. And your conversations will be a LOT more fun.

If you're wearing a coat and sweater in the bar, and a woman asks why you have so many layers on... the safe thing to say is, "I'm cold." Instead, you say something like, "I'm just trying to cover up my insecurities."

Instead of, "Oh, you're from Georgia? Cool!" you can say, "Damn, woman. Southern Belles make my heart ring. This is perfect for me."

You make sexual jokes and innuendos without holding back for fear of disapproval.

Don't just do this with words, though. If you want to kiss a woman, go for it. If she rejects you, shrug it off and go for the kiss ten minutes later. See what happens.

When you filter yourself, you're concerned with the woman's reaction. You walk on eggshells, hoping you don't do anything she doesn't approve of. You're not being genuine.

When women tell you to "be yourself," they want the "unfiltered you" who doesn't hold back. Not the 'polite' you who seeks their approval.

Silence your inner critic. Tell the awkward joke. Go for the kiss at the wrong time. Make things sexual. Live a little. Your conversations will flow, and you'll make deeper connections.

Chapter 12:

Fear of Rejection

I f we want to start a conversation with a woman, the first thing we should do is approach her and start talking. Now, the reality is that most men suffer from anxiety over approaching her, so they often fail to do it.

That's the moment when we try to force ourselves to start a conversation with a woman and then start thinking of thousands of random reasons not to do so: "What if I'm too fat?", "and if I'm not on her level?", "and if she thinks I'm a loser?", "and if my biceps aren't sculpted enough?".

We over-analyze the situation in a way that paralyzes us. "I'm not ready yet," we think. We still need to read a little more, we tell ourselves. However, if we suddenly start talking to a woman and have a good time, none of those thoughts matter anymore. We begin to relax and enjoy ourselves. We realize that we don't need to know anything else about seduction and that this book is unnecessary (careful!).

While we might think that all those fears and insecurities in our minds are relevant and valid, the truth is that they don't matter at all. We just have to go and talk to her. It sounds simple, but I know that sometimes it can be very difficult.

And What If She Rejects Us?

There will be moments when all you get is a completely negative response. Something like: I'm busy, go away! I have a boyfriend! I like women! Sorry, I'm going to become a nun!" or whatever other type of rejection can happen to you.

Let's not let that rejection affect us. I know many people who give it a lot of importance when they get rejected as if it had some real meaning. The only thing they are doing is avoiding true learning by saving themselves the discomfort of that "no." She doesn't know us, and there may be thousands of reasons why she doesn't want to be with us, such as, "your biceps aren't sculpted enough."

The truth is that we often judge rejection from our own metrics and insecurities. Men tell themselves, "I'm sure she rejected me because I'm ugly," "my hair doesn't look good," "I'm not that important," "my shoes are not Nike," etc. Stupid stuff. Their reasons for rejecting us may be very different from those we imagine, but we shouldn't care at all.

Why?

Because her opinion shouldn't affect our life. If we think that she is right and we don't like something about our condition, we should work to change or improve it, not victimize ourselves and cry about it.

I've spent years in the area of seduction, and I've received hundreds of rejections, probably many more than anyone who is reading this book. I admit that some have hurt me, either because of inexperience or being unjustly attacked.

I remember one night when I had already been a coach for a few months, I saw a woman sitting in a club, and I sat next to her. I'm not sure if I was able to say anything, but if I had, it was something really trivial. She looked at me with the face of a rabid dog, almost as if she was barking and foam was spewing out of her mouth while insulting and repudiating me. I ran out of there with my tail between my legs, and I couldn't approach any other woman that night; the feeling was horrible.

I've had very few rejections like that, and nowadays, they don't mean anything to me. I barely think that I had anything to do with her rejecting me like that. She probably had a bad day, maybe she just had a bad break-up with her boyfriend, or she could have lost a loved one. Maybe she didn't like my face, but why should I care?

Another night I was in a bar in Singapore. I saw a tall and very attractive woman in her 20s. She probably would have intimidated me a lot when I'd just started in the art of seduction, and I wouldn't have believed that any of my openers would work, but by that time, I wasn't a rookie.

I approached her, saying "hello!" with a smile. She looked at me smiling without saying anything and turned away. Behind me, one of her much shorter friends with glasses appeared as if she were her henchman. She was pretty cute herself, but the contrast with the other woman did not favor her. "You're not in her league," she exclaimed, going behind her friend. I laughed without caring. That time was the first time that my rejection was announced by somebody else.

Now I'm telling this story because there are going to be ridiculous, absurd, and funny rejections. Failures are nothing, but experiences and a life full of experiences is a richer life. Whether they are good or bad experiences will always depend on our way of looking at them and what we learn.

When approaching a woman, we should always assume that she is attracted to us, although, of course, this is not always the case. Most women will not be available or interested in us. However, if we assume that they are, it will make it easier to approach them and even to get rejected... I mean, they're the ones missing out anyway.

Never pretend that approaches are perfect. Many times they are disorderly, improvised, unpredictable, clumsy, stupid, or ridiculous. Let's embrace randomness and disorder, accept that they will never be perfect, and just get close to her!

If she rejects us, we can simply move on to the next woman until we find someone we match up well with. Most people tend to take rejections personally, which is a way to see everything that others say about us as something real.

Do not expect everyone to accept you.

First Impressions

Studies show that we generate a large amount of our perception of other people in the first few minutes of meeting them. This first perception can still have an influence even through the first weeks or months of a relationship. As Oscar Wilde put it: "You never get a second chance to make a first impression."

However, a big mistake is believing that people's first impressions of us are based on what we say. The truth is that most people don't remember what the first words were but the presence, look, emotional need, and so on. This is another reason why we shouldn't worry so much about "what" to say.

I admit that all this thinking was a bit of a revolution for me at the time. I was a great follower of the openers, pre-set phrases, canned material, or whatever you want to call it. But I remember that everything changed when I start to approach it differently.

Openers can work, but in the long run, I think they end up being a bad choice. In my experience, and in what I've seen in other guys, the more we strive to say the "best phrase," the more we'll end up looking "weird" or "needy." It's not only that what we say may not be in context, but the simple fact that we're looking for a phrase to make her like us makes us seem needier.

In contrast, saying "hello" and presenting yourself in an honest, open way in most cases has a positive or neutral reception. It's simple, and it's natural. So what better starter than that?

Now, if you get a lot of rejections by saying "hello" and introducing yourself, it may be because:

- You present yourself poorly (Negative body language, poorly dressed, acting needy, little eye contact, etc.)

- You approach for the wrong reasons. If you do it looking to impress your friends, expecting a reaction from the other person, or even as if the woman is just another notch on the bedpost, then your reasons are wrong. On the other hand, if you approach a woman that you like and you say she is cute because you really think that, then you are doing it the right way.

With the fact that you've gotten to speak with her for just a moment, you've started off on the right foot. Next, it will depend on your ability to have an exciting conversation.

The Three-Second Rule

One of the best ways to overcome the anxiety of the approach is the three-second rule. This rule consists of going to talk to a woman within a period of 3 seconds, counting from the moment when we first see her. Our brain does not have time to process what it is doing correctly, and we get to her before it selfsabotages. This rule can be very powerful, but it is not perfect because it also takes time to get used to doing it.

The idea is to avoid standing like a dog next to a woman trying to convince us to talk to her. Applying the rule, I think, will give her a good first impression of us because it shows great security even if we start stuttering without knowing what to say.

But the truth is that the three-second rule is often difficult to apply because we don't know what to say. It makes no sense to get so invested in what phrase you need to start a conversation because, as I said before, it is irrelevant.

When I first arrived in Australia, one of the first countries I had ever visited, my English was more like a Tarzanic dialect than anything else. I practically hit my chest with my fists to communicate. During my first two months living in Australia, every time I approached a woman and tried to tell her, "I like you," I would say "you like me," which, despite my mistake, led to the interaction beginning with a smile on her part. Many times the woman would correct me, but sometimes I confused their words and did not care. After that, the conversation flowed...

If she likes you, she'll be willing to listen. On the other hand, if you don't interest her, not even the most ingenious phrase will be enough. As I said before, attraction usually happens long before you say the first word.

Another good methodology to implement is to start talking with three groups of different women in the first half-hour in a bar or club. The important thing is to get yourself completely wet, like the analogy of jumping into a pool. Every time we are about to jump into a pool with a temperature we are not used to, we are bothered by even the slightest splash. But after we jump into it a few times, we start to get used to it and enjoy ourselves. The same happens with approach anxiety. The first woman we talk to in a pub (or anywhere for that matter) may make us feel uncomfortable or uneasy, and it may always be so, but once we are in the game, it starts being fun. So, if you want to write your own story, go out and get splashed!

Chapter 13:
Lessons of Chivalry

I want to establish that being a real gentleman is so much more than dressing accordingly. While dress code inevitably carries a lot of importance, the key to becoming a better version of yourself is educating your mental state and behavior. It's not difficult to comprehend why I'm saying this, as, even though you were to be the best-dressed man in the room, and your attitude wouldn't portray that of a gentleman, it would be all for nothing.

Let's establish one primary thing. Chivalry is not old-fashioned and will never be. The exact measure that indicates a man's value is respect towards himself and others, which is portrayed through chivalry.

Appreciatively, our society has made substantial progress concerning gender equality. Thankfully, the days in which women were perceived as property and inferior to men are gone. But, with this main advantage came a crucial side effect, which has made chivalry quite a problematic aspect. Gender equality causes the greater majority of men to treat women as if they were men. Even though it is crystal clear that men and women are equals, that doesn't mean you should treat a woman the same as you would a man. While this aspect is quite debatable, taking into account the modern-day context, the truth is that every woman, deep inside, wants to be truly respected and treated like a lady.

Besides still having a prominent place in our contemporary society, it's also important to understand that being a gentleman also knows no age. A chivalrous attitude is a desirable trait for all men and boys in any age group.

You can thus teach your young child from an early age that being a gentleman is important. Make sure he understands that girls are different and that he shouldn't treat them how he would treat the rest of the boys his age. It helps a great deal if he has a sister of similar age, whom he can learn to respect, protect, and help from early on. This will serve to shape his worldview and make him adopt the right attitude for later in life. You'd be surprised by how much of our character is built and predetermined in our early childhood.

Of course, another crucial stage of life is the teens. This is where a young man's personality begins to become more consolidated, and all that he has learned up to that point plays an important part in shaping the kind of man he turns into. For most boys, it's also the age of crushing after girls and starting to get involved in relationships. The interactions between men and women change rapidly through different stages of life, and the aspects of gentlemanly conduct do as well. Girls at different ages also expect different things from boys and men.

It's unlikely that a teenager will be able to take his girlfriend out to a fancy dinner or the like, so it's about the little things at this age. Showing small acts of affection and respect like holding doors for women, giving them his jacket when it's cold, and other small gestures like those are what make a teenage boy stand out as a gentleman in the making. The attitude develops from there on if fostered, and the teenager will grow into a man who respects women all his life.

A real gentleman never ceases to be such, though, not even in old age. By that time, he will have long found his companion in life and will have learned all her quirks and beauties, marking him as an expert on making her happy. There isn't all that much learning left to do at that point either, particularly when it comes to being a gentleman. A man that has maintained a happy marriage and carried it on into his late years is a doctor in the field anyway. As you will notice with many elderly men, they are always kind and pleasant towards women they come into contact with during their day, regardless of their age.

Let's see some of the main principles a gentleman should live by.

Treat Everyone with Genuine Respect

I want to outline that a gentleman isn't respectful only to the women he is interested in. On the contrary, a gentleman is an individual who is actually attentive to other men, elderly fellows, and children as well. If you wish to adopt the attitude of a gentleman as a means to get a woman to like you, this isn't right! Such an attitude isn't something you turn on and off as you please, this would make you a hypocrite, and that's the last thing you want.

This may not be the first thing to occur to you, but being a gentleman has quite an important place in the interactions among men as well. Obviously, it's not about catering to their needs per se because it works a little differently in male circles.

Carrying yourself gentlemanly with other men means adhering to a few basic principles, most of which relate to sportsmanship, honor, camaraderie, and empathy. First and foremost, being a gentleman means not taking cheap shots at your opponents in any setting or circumstances. If you are competing for a promotion, for instance, it wouldn't be very chivalrous to sabotage your competition and employ other dirty tactics to get ahead. A gentleman also doesn't kick a man while he's down, neither literally nor figuratively. If you have differences with someone, don't jump the opportunity to get revenge as soon as they fall on hard times and things don't go their way. Raveling in another's failure and taking advantage whenever an opportunity presents itself is very lowly and unbecoming of a gentleman.

Furthermore, I don't know if I even have to state something as obvious, but a gentleman will never, under any circumstances, bully someone and prey on the weaker. There is no world in which this behavior is excusable and anything but an offense against basic human dignity. As a matter of fact, not only will a gentleman never bully someone weaker than him, he will even stand up for those who fall victim to bullies. Another thing that follows up on bullying and mistreatment of the weak, which a gentleman doesn't do, is the abuse of power and position in general. Using a position of influence as a means for personal gain or simply using it to exert power on others just for the sake of exerting power is highly unethical and dishonorable, to say the least.

And last but definitely not least, a gentleman doesn't start a fight. However, yet another difference between a gentleman and a guy who is merely nice is that a gentleman won't run away from a confrontation either. Of course, he will avoid unnecessary conflict, especially a physical one, if he can, but he won't do so at all costs. A real gentleman will be the kind of guy who doesn't look for trouble and can defuse almost any situation, which is why gentlemen rarely get into fights, if ever. However, life can throw you into a situation where the only alternative to getting into a confrontation is to compromise your very dignity, which a gentleman will never do. As a particular popular song has to say on the subject, "A gentleman will walk but never run."

As you have learned so far, though, it's crucial to be chivalrous in simpler ways and with little things that can happen every day if you are to project yourself as a gentleman all the time, not just in critical situations. Now, I would like to start with the basic rules of chivalry.

The Magic Of "Thank You," "Please," And "Excuse Me"

These basic yet essential phrases are more than crucial in outlining your character and respect towards the people you get in contact with. The use of these phrases can go a long way in helping you deliver the right impression.

Using "thank you" indicates your genuine gratitude towards the person who has helped you in a way or another. Also, "please" is the magical phrase that proves you are attentive and considerate of other people. Of course, "excuse me" is an equally powerful word combo that has imperial power. Every time you accidentally get into someone on the street or at work, you shouldn't hesitate to say, "excuse me." This also applies to situations when you need to leave the room or the table, especially when you're on a date!

What you get in exchange for using these everyday phrases is also important. More often than not, a nice word or two will open many doors for you. Most people are likely to be disarmed by such an approach, especially if it's coupled with a sincere smile, and it will be more difficult for them to be rude towards an individual who treats them well. Counter workers, for example, and employees in any sort of administration that deals with a lot of people daily are known for being some of the most frustrated individuals you can run into. If you approach them with a poor attitude, it will only make the interaction even more unpleasant. If you are well-mannered, on the other hand, they are likely to be nicer to you in return. Why get into unnecessary altercations that could potentially ruin your day when you can have a pleasant chat instead? Who knows, your manners and smile may even change someone's day for the better.

Don't Wait to Open Doors

After reading this, you might say – why should I be opening doors? It's not like I'm an usher or something? But, believe it or not, holding the door open, to some women, is definitely an attractive quality. Still, bear in mind that while some women may convey this gesture as lovely, others may find it inappropriate. For this reason, always ask before opening the door for someone. Only ask, "May I hold the door for you?" According to the answer you receive, you will know what to do next.

Give Up Your Seat

Whenever you are traveling using public transport, always pay attention to elderly citizens, pregnant women, or women in general. If the place is packed, and you see a person struggling to stay on their feet, I would recommend you take the attitude of a real gentleman and offer your seat. You don't have to act unnatural, only ask a simple question such as "can I offer you my seat?" Such a simple gesture will speak for your character, and it goes a long way ahead of you.

The same goes for people holding babies or having small children with them. A gentleman is nice to kids, and people generally hold those who are good to children in very high regard. I can hardly think of anything less gentlemanly than a guy sitting and staring out through the window while someone next to him is struggling with a kid or few on a crowded train or a bus.

Conclusion

T alking to women can be tricky. When should you make eye contact? When should you speak? Should you use your inside voice? What are some topics that are popular with women?

What should you do when you are talking to a woman? What is proper etiquette when it comes to women? Here are they, in summary:

Eye contact: Make sure your eyes match the strength of your spine. Be courageous! Make eye contact and hold it for at least three seconds (longer if possible). If you manage a six-second gaze, she will surely swoon! If a man cannot look his woman in the eyes, how can he be expected to look her... elsewhere? Eye contact is important because it lets the lady know that you are paying attention and that she has your permission to continue speaking.

Speaking: the most important part of your communication should come from the mouth. Using your mouth can be difficult for some, so have a few rehearsed lines ready to go! "What's up?" is always a good choice and shows that you are an active listener. Another good choice is "How are you?" When she responds, nod to show that you heard her. Don't just nod because she's cute though, nod because it shows that you care about what she has to say! Nodding will also give her the impression that you agree with what she says; this will make her feel more comfortable.

Sometimes you'll have to say something original, but it's okay. "Nice weather we're having" is always a good choice.

Body language: before approaching, take off your hat and hold it by the brim (this is important). While approaching the woman, stand straight and make sure there are no wrinkles in your shirt. Also, look at her face! This will let her know that you're paying attention and that she has your full permission to continue speaking. When you speak with women, try to keep your hands out of your pockets. It makes them feel uncomfortable because they wonder if you are hiding something (your hand or other body parts). If they ask what you have in your pocket, tell them.

As we end this book, I would like to point out once more the important guidelines:

1. The one thing you need to realize is that women, in general, have been hit on way too much by guys who put more emphasis on the clothes she was wearing than her personality.

2. Even if she's dressed like a bag lady, give her a chance and get past the exterior - there may be something underneath that will make you want to hit up on her.

3. There are three kinds of women: those who will never go out with you, those who will go out with you if you ask them, and those who would ask YOU out if given the chance. The trick is figuring out which one she is before you ask her!

4. Don't be offended if a woman says "no." Maybe you've misread the signs. At times, women just need to be "real" with someone, so they end up shooting you an angry look when you approach them.

5. Don't let the fact that she's ignoring your attempt at winning her over stop you from trying! Be confident and positive! I'm sure that one day in the future, she'll be seeing your name at the top of a list of people she wants to go out with!

6. And lastly...don't get discouraged. The majority of times, women want to be approached by a guy they find attractive. The saying goes: "What's not to like?"

And that's the end of this book. I'd like to thank all of my readers for their support and interest in this book - it was a lot of fun writing it.